FIGHTING CANCER

FIGHTING **CANCER**

BY THE EDITORS OF TIME-LIFE BOOKS

LIBRARY OF HEALTH / TIME-LIFE BOOKS / ALEXANDRIA, VIRGINIA

THE CONSULTANT:

Dr. David Schottenfeld is Chief of Epidemiology and Preventive Medicine at the Memorial Sloan-Kettering Cancer Center in New York City. He is also Professor of Public Health at Cornell University Medical College, where he received his M.D. degree in 1956.

For information about any Time-Life book, please write:
Reader Information, Time-Life Books,
541 North Fairbanks Court, Chicago, Illinois 60611.

Library of Congress Cataloguing in Publication Data
The Editors of Time-Life Books
    Fighting Cancer
    (Library of Health)
    Bibliography: p.
    Includes index.
    1. Cancer   I. Time-Life Books.   II. Series.
RC263.F48   616.99'4   81-8799
ISBN 0-8094-3764-3
ISBN 0-8094-3763-5 (lib. bdg.)
ISBN 0-8094-3762-7 (retail ed.)

LIBRARY OF HEALTH

Editorial Staff for *Fighting Cancer*
Editor: William Frankel
Assistant Editor: Phyllis K. Wise
Designer: Albert Sherman
Picture Editor: Jane N. Coughran
Text Editors: Lee Hassig, C. Tyler Mathisen, Paul N. Mathless
Staff Writers: Laura Longley Babb, Roger E. Herst, Peter Kaufman, John Newton
Researchers: Norma E. Kennedy, James Robert Stengel (principals), Janet Doughty, Judy D. French, Carlos Vidal Greth Barbara Hicks, Rita Thievon Mullin, Trudy W. Pearson
Assistant Designer: Cynthia T. Richardson
Editorial Assistant: Nana Heinbaugh Juarbe
Special Contributors: Oliver Allen, Susan Perry Dawson, Norman Kolpas, Patricia Molino, Wendy Murphy, David S. Thomson, Gene Thornton, Edmund White

EDITORIAL PRODUCTION
Production Editor: Douglas B. Graham
Operations Manager: Gennaro C. Esposito, Gordon E. Buck (assistant)
Assistant Production Editor: Feliciano Madrid
Quality Control: Robert L. Young (director), James J. Cox (assistant), Daniel J. McSweeney, Michael G. Wight (associates)
Art Coordinator: Anne B. Landry
Copy Staff: Susan B. Galloway (chief), Margery duMond, Sheirazada Hann, Celia Beattie
Picture Department: Renée DeSandies
Traffic: Kimberly K. Lewis

Correspondents: Elisabeth Kraemer, Helga Kohl (Bonn); Margot Hapgood, Dorothy Bacon, Lesley Coleman (London); Susan Jonas, Lucy T. Voulgaris (New York); Maria Vincenza Aloisi, Josephine du Brusle (Paris); Ann Natanson (Rome). Valuable assistance was also given by: Robert Kroon (Geneva); Lance Keyworth (Helsinki); Peter Hawthorne (Johannesburg); Judy Aspinall, Jeremy Lawrence, Karin B. Pearce, Pippa Pridham (London); Felix Rosenthal (Moscow); Marcia Gauger (New Delhi); Carolyn T. Chubet, Miriam Hsia, Christina Lieberman (New York); Mimi Murphy (Rome); Mary Johnson (Stockholm); Edwin Reingold, Eiko Fukuda, Frank Iwama, Keiko Nagasaka (Tokyo).

CONTENTS

CHAPTER 1

Victories over a dread disease

The many cancers that can be prevented
How malignancy begins
A universal plague in many guises
Who falls victim and why
Tracking killers in the laboratory
Triumphs of treatment
The worldwide army of cancer fighters

"Cancer," wrote Dr. Vincent DeVita, Director of America's National Cancer Institute, in 1980, "is one of the most curable chronic diseases in this country today."

The statement may seem surprising. If any disease has the reputation of being incurable, it is cancer. The very word has had the force of an epitaph, a synonym for death. For centuries—and in some places, even today—victims were not told the name of their disease. Families refused to acknowledge the presence of cancer in their midst, even after fathers, mothers or children had succumbed, and newspaper obituary writers sidestepped the dreaded word with a common euphemism: death "after a long illness." These bitter heritages of aversion and fear are becoming meaningless. In sober truth, Dr. DeVita's apparently bold claim is reality today. It is a claim based largely upon the rate of improvement in "five-year survival"—the period after diagnosis when, if the patient is kept free of symptoms, most types of cancers are considered cured. For most common types of cancer, this rate jumped spectacularly in the decades between World War II and the end of the 1970s. The change in the statistics over this period is little short of miraculous:

● For cancer of the colon, the five-year survival rate rose from about 32 per cent to nearly 49 per cent.

● Among women suffering from breast cancer, barely one out of two formerly survived for five years; a generation later more than two out of three recovered.

● For prostate cancer the rate went up from 37 per cent to nearly 63 per cent.

● Cancer of the bladder had a 42 per cent five-year survival rate; the rate climbed to 61 per cent.

● Five-year survival for cancer of the cervix, or mouth of the womb, rose from 47 per cent to 64 per cent; for cancers within the womb, from 61 per cent to 81 per cent.

● Hodgkin's disease, a cancer of the body's infection-fighting system, was practically conquered: The cure rate rose from a dismal 25 per cent to a heartening 67 per cent.

● The most common type of acute leukemia, a cancer of the blood-forming tissues so virulent that all victims used to die within months after its detection, was made curable for 28 per cent of its victims.

Underlying such specific examples are the overall figures for cancer cure. In the 1930s, 25 per cent of all those stricken by cancer in the United States were treated and cured. By 1955 the figure was up to 33 per cent. By 1980 medical scientists estimated that among those who developed all types of cancer, 58 per cent could be cured, with a life expectancy equal to that of someone who had never been stricken at all.

These triumphs of treatment are only part of the story. It now is possible not only to cure a wide variety of cancers, but to prevent many of the types that are difficult to cure. Lung cancer is an outstanding example of a deadly, essentially preventable cancer. More men in the industrialized world suffer from it than from any other type, aside from easily curable skin cancers. Among women, it is increasing faster than any other type of cancer. Because lung cancer is usually far advanced when first detected, its overall cure rate remains

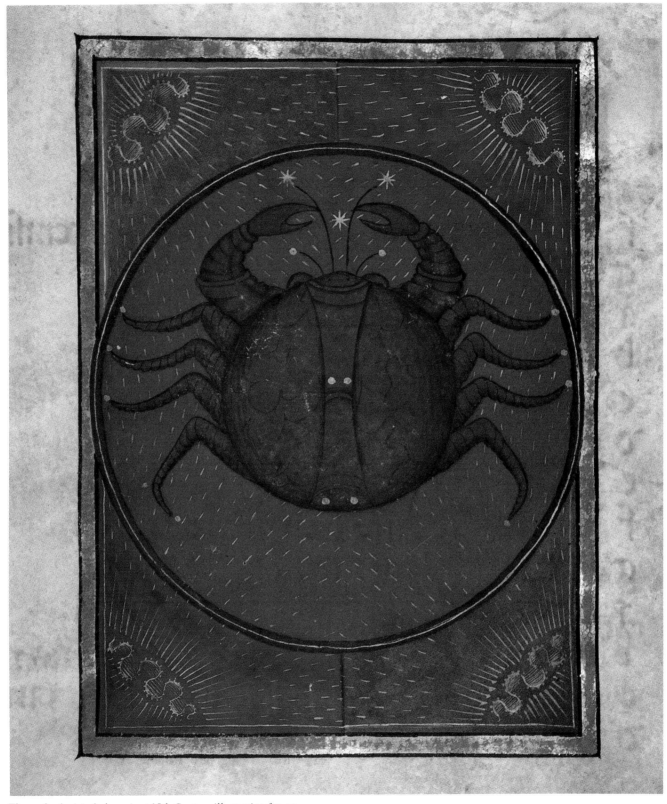

The crab, depicted above in a 15th Century illustration for an
Italian book of prayers, gave mankind's dreaded disease its name.
The hard center and clawlike projections of a spreading tumor
seemed to Hippocrates, the ancient-Greek physician, to resemble
the crustacean, and he named the disease ''karkinoma,'' after
the Greek word for ''crab.'' ''Cancer'' is the Latin translation.

low: about 10 per cent. But much of it is easy to prevent—and not getting it in the first place is better than any cure. The villain, of course, is smoking. Heavy smokers are 20 times more likely to develop lung cancer than nonsmokers. In a country such as the United States, where lung cancer is common, the implications are clear. If the last cigarette in the United States were smoked today, the rate of lung-cancer attacks would drop from 56 to 14 per 100,000 in 30 years.

The many cancers that can be prevented

Smoking is only one among many avoidable causes of cancer. Alcohol is another; so are certain foods, and certain substances added to foods to preserve or flavor them. Overexposure to the sun's radiation can produce a skin cancer, and the penetrating radiation of X-rays can cause cancers deep in the body. Most insidious and diverse of all are the cancer-causing chemicals encountered in factories, mines and almost every other area in which materials are processed or chemically changed. Hardly a month passes in which cancer detectives do not identify a new suspect for this rogues' gallery or find a new outbreak of a known criminal.

Substances and forces that cause cancer are called carcinogens. The hunt for them goes on, and campaigns to eradicate them are only beginning to have an effect. But if every carcinogen now recognized could be eliminated overnight, the incidence of cancer would be cut in half by the year 2000.

It is in the light of such hard facts that Dr. Vincent DeVita's statement on cancer's curability assumes its full dimensions. Half of all cancers can be prevented; more than half of those that cannot be prevented can be cured. Over the next generation, because of these two facts alone, the annual number of cancer deaths in the industrialized world can be reduced from 183 to 55 per 100,000. The estimate is conservative; further—and almost certain—advances in prevention and cure would improve it. Clearly, the war against cancer is winnable, and it is being won.

The war is far from over. Cancer remains a major killer: In the United States, it takes about 390,000 lives a year; in England, 122,000; in West Germany, 155,000; in the Soviet Union, 360,000—the worldwide figure may be a staggering four million. On many fronts, campaigns against the disease falter or do not move at all. Avoiding carcinogens in everyday life means giving up cherished habits; eliminating them from the workplace has heavy economic consequences—lost jobs, lost revenues and increased costs. Early detection and diagnosis, which offer the best chance of curing a cancer, are often neglected or ignored; and some types of cancer still stubbornly resist the best available treatments.

The battles that have been won in the desperate war on cancer are almost entirely victories of recent years. Until the end of the 19th Century, the disease was indeed essentially incurable; some superficial cancers could be removed by surgery, but nothing more. At the turn of the 20th the range of therapy broadened to include X-ray treatments, which can burn away both surface and deep cancers; the nature and causes of the disease, however, were still matters of speculation. Then, with the explosive growth of medical knowledge following World War II, scientists and physicians acquired four major resources in their unending battle, all new and all further strengthened with each passing year. They know how to prevent most cancers. They have superb diagnostic tools to catch it early, often long before any ordinary symptoms of illness appear. They have an arsenal of marvelously effective weapons against it—treatments by surgery, radiation and drugs that far surpass anything the world has ever known. And perhaps most important, they know what cancer is.

How malignancy begins

Cancer had been such a dark and fearful mystery because it takes so many forms. It can strike any organ, any tissue, anywhere in the body. But despite this diversity, all cancers share certain characteristics. They are all diseases of individual cells, the basic building blocks of plants and animals.

No multicelled organism is immune to these diseases. A growth called crown gall, which appears on a number of plants, including daisies and tomatoes, exhibits certain characteristics of cancer. Insects get cancer; the fruit fly, a favorite creature of experimenters because it reproduces so rapidly—more than 35 generations per year—suffers from both brain tumors and blood cancers. Fish that swim through harbors polluted by tars and oil that cause cancer in human beings develop cancers similar to human cancer. Dogs, cats, cows and horses get cancers of various types. Some wild animals, such as cheetahs and certain Asiatic bears, were once thought to be immune. They are not. Protected in a laboratory or a zoo from disease and their natural enemies, so that they consistently reach an age old for their species, they too develop the disease.

In all of these living things, a cancer starts when something goes awry inside a cell, the smallest unit of living tissue. An error is somehow introduced into the genetic code, the complex pattern of molecules that normally ensures the reproduction of a new cell perfectly fitted to its function in the body. The genetic error may be caused by a chemical; by radiation, such as that of the sun or of X-rays; or by the tiny agents of disease called viruses. In addition, many genetic disruptions are simply random slippages of the cell's machinery, with no discernible cause. The result is the same: a new-born freak cell called a mutant.

Few mutant cells survive long enough to do any damage. Some are so deformed or deficient that they wither and die; others are destroyed by the body's natural defenses. In a cancer victim, however, at least one such cell hangs on to life and eludes the body's defenders. The cell divides into two, the two into four. Eventually, a billion or more may form a tumor—a swollen lump perceptible to the touch.

Rarely do swellings indicate the growth of new tissue, and even more rarely are they dangerous. The hard knot that follows a bump on the head is simply an accumulation of fluid beneath the skin; other swellings are caused by pus at the site of an infection. Even a tumor consisting of mutant cells is seldom cancerous; most tumorous lumps are classified as benign and generally can be ignored. Only malignant, or cancerous, tumors inevitably pose a threat to life.

The two types of tumors differ in a variety of ways. A benign tumor—the wart is a familiar example—is almost always enclosed in a capsule or sheath of fibrous tissue. Malignant tumors are rarely so well confined, and tend to invade adjacent tissues. Some exceptions to this rule do exist. Wilms' tumor, for example, a cancer that strikes at the

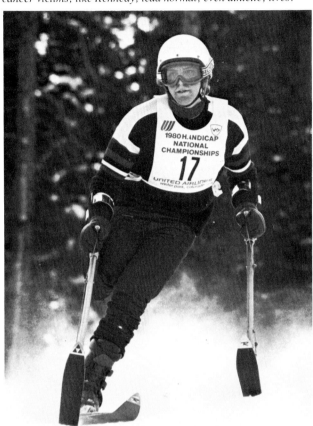

Six years after the amputation of his cancerous right leg, Ted Kennedy Jr., son of the U.S. Senator from Massachusetts, competes in a ski race, using one regular ski and, for balance, "outriggers" made from short skis on poles. With such devices to help compensate for lost limbs or organs, more and more cancer victims, like Kennedy, lead normal, even athletic, lives.

kidneys in children, is encapsulated, like a benign growth.

When the outward appearance of a tumor does not reveal its nature, the distinction between benign and malignant can be seen through a microscope. If a kidney tumor is benign, the cells within it closely resemble those of the kidney itself, in patterning and structure. In Wilms' tumor—and in all other cancerous tumors—the cells have only a rough resemblance to those of the tissues in which they originally grew. Instead, they take on characteristics of their own. A normal cell has a single small body, the nucleus, at its center; a cancer cell may have a huge nucleus, or two or more nuclei. Like the nucleus, other components of the cell's interior may be deformed or multiplied. An entire cancer cell is usually misshapen, and groups of them grow helter-skelter, lacking the orderly arrangements of normal cells.

There is a third difference between the two types of tumor—the most important distinction of all. Benign tumors are localized; they grow, generally quite slowly, but they stay at their original sites. Cancer tumors establish outposts elsewhere in the body, by a process called metastasis.

Benign tumors can be harmful despite their name. A small benign tumor inside the skull may block the blood supply to the brain, causing a stroke. Larger tumors can be dangerous anywhere in the body—and benign tumors weighing 70 pounds have been recorded. A medium-sized or large tumor can deform vital organs and interfere with their functions.

Malignant tumors can have the same effects, but their real menace lies in metastasis. The process begins when a cancer cell breaks away from the tumor. The malignant cell may enter the bloodstream and be swept to a distant site almost anywhere in the body. Wherever this wandering parasite comes to rest, it is dangerous. "What no normal cell is capable of," wrote the French cancer researcher Dr. Lucien Israël, "every cancer cell can do. It grows, regardless of local conditions, and its descendants reproduce more or less crudely the tissue from which it came. Thus fragments of intestine, bone or stomach will be found in the lung."

The bloodstream is only one of the pathways of propagation. Cells from a malignant tumor may be absorbed directly by a clear, watery fluid called lymph that is conveyed throughout the body by a network of lymphatic vessels. The malignant cells picked up by lymph may then lodge in filter-like structures called lymph nodes *(pages 106-107)*. (Ironically, the lymphatic system normally serves to protect the body against disease.) Malignant cells can even work their way through solid tissue; a cancer in the lining of the stomach, for example, can grow through the stomach wall to establish colonies elsewhere in the abdominal cavity.

It is after metastasis that cancer is most deadly. Thousands of individual cells or microscopic tumors may lie hidden in the body and, as Dr. Ronald Glasser of the University of Minnesota wrote, "each and every one must be hunted down and killed. If just one is left anywhere, it will grow again and

again, until it finally wins." Having grown, a cancer may take over an artery, blocking the flow of blood to such vital organs as the kidneys, liver and heart. Cancer in the pancreas or the bone marrow may reduce the blood's ability to clot; if internal bleeding begins elsewhere in the body—possibly from a blood vessel ruptured by a metastasized tumor—the victim may die of it. Cancer colonies in the lymphatic system so weaken the body's defenses that an ordinary fungus infection, usually simple and easy to cure, will rage out of control.

Of all cancer's effects, the best known and most disturbing may be a pattern of symptoms called cachexia. It begins with an inexplicable loss of appetite. Weight drops off—sometimes slowly, sometimes with frightening speed—muscles become weak, sleep elusive. Pain is constant. As the malnourished body deteriorates, wastes within it reach toxic levels. Eventually the victim goes into a deep, terminal coma.

A universal plague in many guises

Such are the ravages of advanced cancer—the ultimate effects of a single diseased cell. The disease is both ancient and universal. Examinations of Egyptian mummies have revealed bone cancer in people who lived 5,000 years ago. The Incan Indians who inhabited Peru 24 centuries ago developed not only bone cancer, but a virulent form of skin cancer called melanoma. Among both peoples, the incidence of the disease was apparently low—only a few cancers have been seen in the thousands of mummies and skeletons that have been studied. The ancient Egyptians and Inca were short-lived peoples; most of them presumably died of other diseases or of injuries long before cancer had time to develop.

In the modern world, no branch of the human family tree is known to be free of cancer, though rumors to the contrary keep popping up. In 1977, for example, the United Nations Educational, Scientific and Cultural Organization reported that the people of Pakistan's remote Hunza Valley showed no signs of the disease. The U.N. report was proved wrong; the Hunzas have insignificantly fewer cases of cancer than other populations of similar size, environment and occupation.

Farmers in the uplands of Soviet Georgia, near the Black Sea, have long been an even richer source of health myth.

They were once said to be not only cancer-free, but even immune to the aging process; tales abounded of people still active at the age of 125. But the accounts of fantastic longevity turned out to be based on provincial chauvinism and bad record-keeping. And the Soviet government, after an intensive study of the Georgians, reported in 1980 that they suffer as much breast, lung and cervical cancer as other Soviet peoples; in fact, only the incidence of stomach and esophageal cancer proved substantially lower than the average.

The facts about the Soviet Georgians illustrate an important truth about cancer: Although the affliction is universal, there are strange variations in its incidence, as a whole and by type. World Health Organization statistics showed that in 1974 and 1975 Scotland had a higher cancer death rate than any other country in the world—more than five and a half times higher than that of Thailand, the country with the fewest cases. Variations among types of cancer were even wider. Japan and Norway had much the same total cancer death rates, but the Japanese suffered three times more stomach cancer than the Norwegians; on the other hand, the death rate from breast cancer among Norwegian women was nearly four times higher than among the women of Japan.

Scientists can explain some of the variations in cancer incidence, including the appalling rate of stomach cancer in Japan. They are virtually certain that the Japanese diet, high in smoked and salted foods and in a known carcinogen called bracken fern, is a major cause of that cancer. Elsewhere, specific cancers have been attributed to specific foods and other agents *(pages 13-15)*. But anomalies and mysteries remain. No one yet knows, for example, why the cancer death rate is highest in Scotland. And no one knows why the breast-cancer death rate is higher in Norway than in Japan, though some scientists have suggested that differences in childbearing or breast-feeding customs may be the key.

Who falls victim and why

To explain why some people get a particular cancer and others do not, or why cancer is more prevalent in one society than in another, medical investigators known as epidemiologists painstakingly compare the dissimilar groups. The tech-

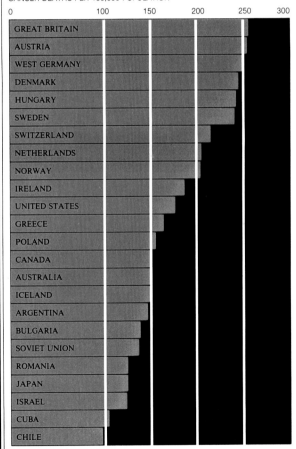

A surprising gamut of vulnerability

Cancer affects all nations, but some more than others. The graph shows death rates from cancer, by number of deaths per 100,000 population, for 24 countries in the late 1970s. A pattern emerges: The rates are generally higher in densely populated and industrialized countries, such as Great Britain and West Germany, and lower in sparsely settled, agrarian or developing nations, such as Canada and Chile. These differences probably come from higher rates of smoking and more exposure to cancer-causing chemicals in urbanized countries and, in developing nations, a lower life expectancy—death comes from other causes before cancer can strike.

niques of epidemiology, based on comparative medical examinations, health records and interviews, have dominated much of 20th Century cancer research, but the seeds of these techniques were planted nearly three centuries ago. In 1700, the Italian doctor Bernardino Ramazzini noted that nuns, who lead lives very different from those of the general population, have a high susceptibility to breast cancer. He concluded—correctly—that it was in some way related to their celibacy.

Among the first to use the techniques was an 18th Century English surgeon, Percivall Pott. A prominent figure in the London of his day, Pott treated such patients as the actor David Garrick and the man of letters Samuel Johnson. He was also a medical scholar, with interests ranging from hernias to broken legs, and in 1775 he turned his attention to a curious phenomenon among London chimney sweeps. At an early age, and to a degree far beyond that of their contemporaries, they were susceptible to cancer of the scrotum.

In "A Short Treatise of the Chimney Sweeper's Cancer," Pott described the work of these boys and young men, "thrust up narrow, and sometimes hot chimnies, where they are bruised, burned, and almost suffocated; and when they get to puberty, become peculiarly liable to a noisome, painful and fatal disease." To get through those narrow chimneys, they often worked naked. They rarely bathed—the practice was considered unhealthful—and soot lay thick upon their skins, especially in the groin area. That soot, Pott pointed out, represented a substance peculiar to the chimney sweeps' trade. In a bold leap of speculation, he declared that the soot was the cause of their cancer.

Pott could never prove his case, but his primitive methods became the foundation of modern cancer epidemiology. This medical specialty now offers the best opportunities for learning what causes cancer in human beings. Like Pott, epidemiologists have linked specific occupations and chemicals to particular cancers; similar studies have implicated diet, sexual habits and heredity as well. In the course of their studies, they have developed two main branches of their science, one essentially retrospective, the other prospective.

Retrospective epidemiologists follow Pott's method, but at a much higher level of thoroughness and sophistication. Having identified a group especially high in a specific cancer or in cancers generally, they probe the lives both of the victims and of those who have escaped the disease. They analyze medical records and personal histories, and the personnel and health records kept by employers. Survivors are questioned on every conceivable detail of their working and living habits, and the investigators search through death certificates to identify earlier cases.

In one typical retrospective project, conducted in 1981, a team of researchers led by Dr. Brian MacMahon of the Harvard School of Public Health studied 369 victims of pancreas cancer and 644 subjects who were free of that cancer. The epidemiologists asked all the subjects about their use of tobacco, alcohol, tea and coffee, in an attempt to discover whether any of these factors increase the risk of developing the disease. One important connection emerged: Pancreas cancer patients were more likely to be coffee drinkers than were the controls. Neither alcohol nor tea increased the risk; cigarette smoking increased it only slightly. What was more, the more coffee a person drank, the greater the risk: Those who drank one or two cups a day were twice as likely to develop pancreas cancer as those who drank no coffee at all; those who drank five or more cups tripled their risk. Obviously, the effects of such a study can be vital to cancer prevention. In the United States, more than half of the population over the age of 10 drinks coffee every day, and Dr. MacMahon estimated that more than half of all pancreas cancer could be linked to coffee drinking.

Unlike Dr. MacMahon, who worked backward from existing records, prospective epidemiologists follow large numbers of people into the future. These people are not necessarily ill when the project starts; the epidemiologist simply records their medical histories and their life styles in great detail, then waits to see what happens to them. The waiting is expensive: Hundreds or even thousands of technicians may keep close track of the subjects for decades. But the findings, based upon identical, exhaustively detailed observations of many people over a long period, are especially valuable.

Perhaps the best known of these elaborate projects is the

Curious pockets of cancer around the world

Cancer plays favorites: Certain forms strike more virulently in certain places. Although most of these geographical concentrations remain to be explained, they often provide clues to a custom or climate that causes the peculiarly local disease.

One form of cancer traced to specific causes, Burkitt's lymphoma *(pages 104-105),* is linked to environment. Six other factors fairly conclusively established as causes of distinctive cancers are illustrated on the following pages. These causes are surprisingly diverse: local foodstuffs or food-preparation techniques, personal habits and a parasite that lives mainly in the Nile River.

Among the most puzzling cancer pockets are those where breast cancer is unusually prevalent. The disease is apparently influenced by many factors—heredity, childbearing, possibly viruses and, according to some authorities, a diet high in fats. None of these suspected causes, however, explains why in all the United States, breast cancer is most common around the Great Lakes.

The concentration of lung cancer in Great Britain and the Southern United States is attributed to cigarette smoking—an almost universal habit—and to industrial pollution in those areas. But no one knows why the states of Georgia and South Carolina should suffer so from esophageal cancer—a widely scattered disease whose suspected causes elsewhere have been isolated. In the Transkei region of South Africa, many Bantu men contract this cancer because, it is speculated, they drink a maize beer that contains a cancer-causing nitrosamine. Alcohol consumption, perhaps in combination with smoking, may be the reason for esophageal cancer in France. And among Iran's nomadic Turkomans, the cause could be their regular fare of sooty bread.

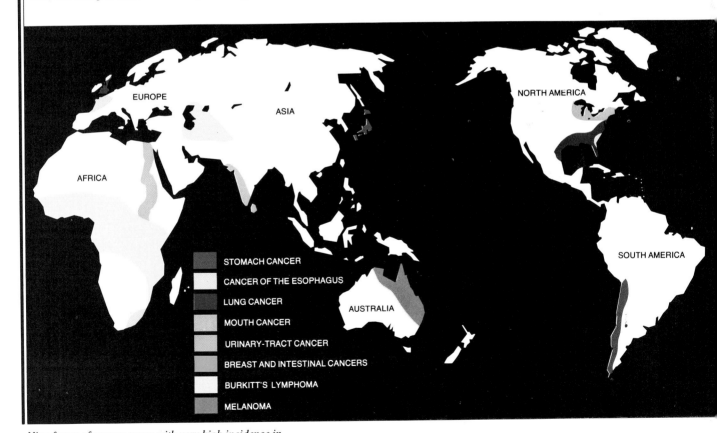

EUROPE
ASIA
AFRICA
NORTH AMERICA
SOUTH AMERICA
AUSTRALIA

STOMACH CANCER
CANCER OF THE ESOPHAGUS
LUNG CANCER
MOUTH CANCER
URINARY-TRACT CANCER
BREAST AND INTESTINAL CANCERS
BURKITT'S LYMPHOMA
MELANOMA

Nine forms of cancer occur with very high incidence in particular places around the globe, a peculiarity that often suggests their causes. Burkitt's lymphoma, a jaw cancer, confined to mosquito-ridden equatorial Africa, is triggered by malaria and other mosquito-borne infections. But in other pockets, causes remain mysterious and cancers overlap.

A Tokyo fish vendor displays the day's offerings of salmon, salmon eggs and codfish eggs, all salted and seasoned with hot peppers. An excess of salt has been linked with stomach cancer; Japan has the world's highest incidence, but pockets of the disease exist wherever salted fish is a staple, as in Chile.

Sunbathing, as on this Queensland beach, is a mania among Australians—most of them fair-skinned and lacking pigment to block the sun's powerful rays. The result is a high rate of skin cancer.

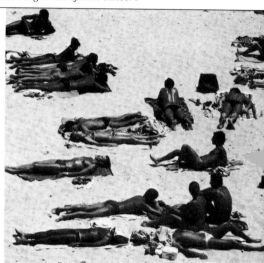

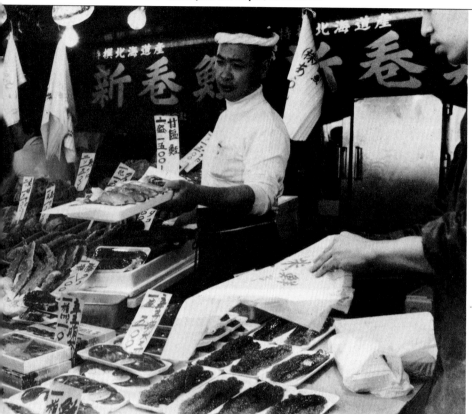

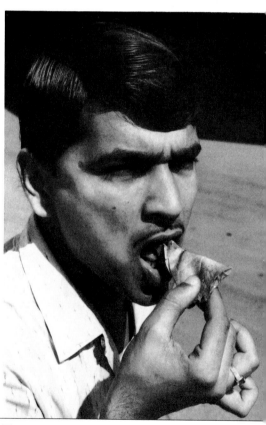

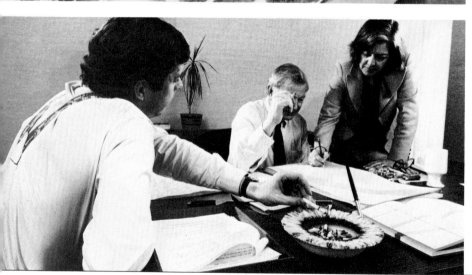

In a scene familiar all over the United States, office workers fill the air—and their lungs—with cigarette smoke. Lung cancer, blamed largely on tobacco, accounts for more than a third of cancer deaths among American men—more than any other cancer— and women's deaths from lung cancer have increased rapidly.

This Indian is eating a betel leaf spread with a paste containing lime, betel nut and tobacco flakes. The juices irritate the mouth, eventually causing cancer. In India, 30 per cent of all cancers are oral.

In her tent in northeastern Iran, a Turkoman woman bakes bread over an open-earth oven. This traditional oven, heated by a fire of scrub bushes, contaminates the bread with soot— a known carcinogen that is thought to cause the cancer of the esophagus so prevalent in this region of the world.

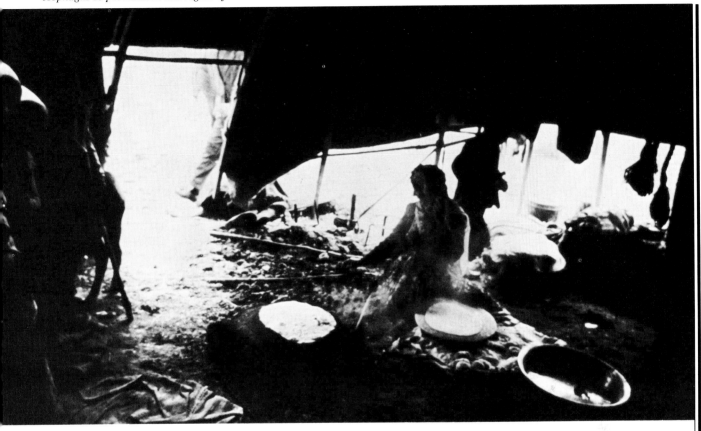

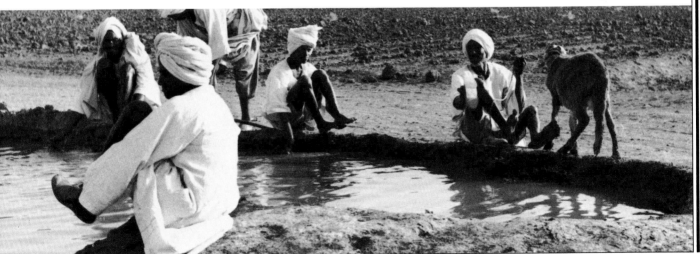

Sudanese wash their feet in a canal near the Nile River, breeding ground of a waterborne, wormlike parasite called schistosome. It enters the urinary tract and lodges in the bladder, causing irritation and inflammation that is blamed for the bladder cancer endemic all along the 4,500-mile river.

Cancer Prevention Study, begun by the American Cancer Society in 1959. At the outset, about one million subjects were chosen by the Society's epidemiologists; a decade and a half later, 800,000 survivors were still under observation. Though the observations covered a variety of medical and personal data, the epidemiologists' objectives were sharply focused: They wanted to compare the lives of subjects who contracted cancer with those who did not, in the hope of identifying hitherto unsuspected causes of the disease and building proof against previously uncertain causes. The experiment proved its value as early as 1964, when the Society showed that cigarette smokers, on the average, had a lung-cancer death rate 10 times higher than that of nonsmokers.

Both retrospective and prospective studies have their limits, some apparent, some real. Neither can prove how a carcinogen causes cancer—but they are not designed to do so. What they reveal, in exact numbers or percentages, is the extent to which a specific agent increases the risk of contracting the disease. The fact that some smokers, for example, never get cancer, while some nonsmokers do, is not in itself a refutation of the Cancer Prevention Study, which claims no more than that smoking increases the odds of getting cancer—or, in the language of epidemiology, that smoking is a "risk factor" for the disease. However, one limitation of such studies is very real. Human beings and their ways of living are almost unreckonably complex and diverse. Identifying a risk factor by epidemiological means alone is difficult at best, unprovable at worst; some other factor, unidentified or underestimated, may be at work.

Tracking killers in the laboratory

Because epidemiological research into the causes of cancer takes so long and may leave crucial questions unanswered, the more direct method of laboratory experimentation is undertaken when possible, as it generally is before the introduction of a newly synthesized chemical into foods or drugs. The two types of techniques often go hand in hand. Some compounds such as soot and certain dyes are known from the findings of epidemiologists to be dangerous. Laboratory tests can identify the components of such compounds that are

to blame—benzopyrene in soot, beta-naphthylamine in dyes—and such tests can also provide indisputable proof that a suspected substance or activity does cause cancer.

When materials suspected as carcinogens are being tested, scientists cannot, of course, risk a human life; laboratory experiments must be done only on animals. During the 1960s, as epidemiological evidence on the risks of smoking began to pour in, generations of mice at the Imperial Cancer Research Fund, in London, panted out their lives in smoke-filled enclosures, and showed evidence of lung cancer. At a Veterans Administration laboratory in New Jersey, in 1970, cigarette smoke was pumped directly into dogs' lungs, through openings cut in their throats, and generated cancerous growths. And in a bizarre experiment of the early 1980s, baboons at the Southwest Research Foundation in San Antonio, Texas, were taught to smoke cigarettes themselves in the continuing quest for hard experimental evidence.

All such trials somewhat resemble a prospective study, in which a scientist selects a group of subjects and follows their course of health or illness. But there is one critical difference. In the laboratory, but not in everyday life, the scientist can be sure that his subjects differ only in the amounts of carcinogen they are exposed to. What they eat, how they exercise or sleep, the very air they breathe—all can be rigidly controlled. Hereditary differences between animals can be reduced or eliminated; among laboratory mice, for example, scientific breeding has produced strains in which all the individuals are genetically identical. Thus, if a scientist exposes one group of mice to a suspected carcinogen, leaving a second group unexposed, and the first group develops cancer while the second does not, he has proved that the substance causes cancer—at least in mice. To move beyond this test, he might repeat it with other animal subjects—rabbits, perhaps, or dogs or monkeys. If a substance induces cancer in several different kinds of mammals, it probably is a carcinogen for most mammals, including human beings.

One of the earliest laboratory trials confirmed the pioneering epidemiological study of Percivall Pott. In 1915, almost a century and a half after Pott published his observations of London chimney sweeps, and in a laboratory on the other side of the globe, two Japanese scientists, Dr. Katsusaburo Yamagiwa and Koichi Ichikawa at the Imperial University in Tokyo, ran tests on the coal tar that was the suspected carcinogen in soot. They painted the tar on the ears of rabbits, and reported that the animals developed a cancer in that area, comparable to the scrotal cancer of the London sweeps.

In modern cancer research the confirmation of a finding is rarely so belated, and practical preventive action can be swift. For vinyl chloride, a chemical used in aerosol sprays and in the manufacture of plastics, epidemiological and laboratory evidence accumulated quickly and simultaneously. In May, 1970, Dr. P. L. Viola, a cancer researcher in Rome, reported that he had developed cancer in animals by using very high doses of the substance, but concluded that the levels encountered in industry presented no danger to workers. Nevertheless, less than two years later American and European chemical manufacturers started both animal tests and epidemiological studies of vinyl chloride.

The first breakthrough came in Italy. In January, 1973, Dr. Cesare Maltoni of Bologna found liver cancers in animals exposed to low levels of the chemical; his experiments were repeated and confirmed by Dr. Viola. Then, in late 1973 and early 1974, three cases of a rare liver cancer turned up at a vinyl chloride plant in Louisville, Kentucky, and an epidemiological search of the death records of workers at other plants showed that the same cancer, often misdiagnosed, had struck again and again. Only a few weeks later, Dr. Maltoni brought in the final damning evidence: He had induced the cancer in his experimental animals, using dosage levels no higher than those faced by the workers in the plants.

As one historian of the episode commented, "people hardly needed any more convincing then." In 1973 and 1974, beginning even before the last pieces of the puzzle had been fitted into place, the use of vinyl chloride in aerosols, which could harm the general public, was banned, and plastics manufacturers reformed their procedures to bring the chemical down to safe levels within their plants.

When the combination of epidemiological and laboratory evidence is as clear-cut as this, the right course of action is equally clear: Scientists, doctors and the news media spread

MEN		WOMEN
2%	BRAIN AND NERVOUS SYSTEM	1%
5%	MOUTH	2%
1%	THYROID	2%
25%	RESPIRATORY SYSTEM	9%
	BREAST	27%
4%	STOMACH	2%
21%	OTHER DIGESTIVE ORGANS	21%
9%	URINARY TRACT	4%
19%	REPRODUCTIVE SYSTEM	19%
3%	BONE, CONNECTIVE TISSUE AND SKIN	2%
3%	LEUKEMIA	3%
5%	OTHER BLOOD AND LYMPH TISSUES	5%
3%	ALL OTHER	3%

HOW CANCER AFFECTS THE SEXES
Most cancers affect men and women equally, as indicated in this chart, which specifies by anatomical area the percentage of all cancers affecting each sex in the United States. Some differences are understandable: Breast cancer strikes mainly women; lung cancer mainly affects men, presumably because men smoke more.

the alarm, and citizens learn to avoid carcinogens they might otherwise inadvertently eat, breathe or touch. In 1976, for example, the people of Montgomery County, Maryland, alerted to the dangers of asbestos dust, forced their highway department to stop covering roads with gravel containing traces of that carcinogen. And throughout the world, men and women have discarded hand-held hair dryers from which asbestos, surrounding the heating elements as insulation, might be blown into the air.

The evidence is not always decisive, and for some substances the risk of exposure must be balanced against real or potential benefits. Consider the case of diethylstilbestrol, or DES, a synthetic hormone that normally helps to make a woman's body a suitable environment for childbearing. From the 1940s to the 1960s many pregnant women received DES as a medicine to prevent miscarriages. Years later, epidemiological studies discovered that the daughters of these women had an abnormally high incidence of cervical and vaginal cancer. The United States government promptly warned pregnant women against using DES as a medicine.

But an official government ruling went further: It also banned the use of DES in cattle feed. Cattle fed small quantities of the hormone gain weight faster; if the DES is omitted from their feed during the last few weeks before slaughtering, only traces of it remain in their bodies, concentrated in the liver. To receive 50 milligrams, the amount in a medicinal dose, a woman would have to eat 25 tons of beef liver. Conceivably, DES might cause cancer in minuscule doses, but such potency has never been seen. Some scientists believe that the benefits from DES-stimulated cattle outweigh the slight risk posed by the carcinogen, and only partly because the cost of the beef is reduced. Ironically, beef from cattle raised on feed completely free of DES carries a slight risk of its own. Such beef is fatter, and cancer of the colon and other organs is somewhat more common in people who eat a diet rich in fat.

The ban on DES was generally accepted, but some risk-versus-benefit controversies have not been resolved. In the 1970s, very large doses of the artificial sweetener saccharin were linked to bladder cancer in a few laboratory animals in studies at the University of Wisconsin, the U.S. Food and Drug Administration and elsewhere, and in 1980 Dr. Robert Hoover of the National Cancer Institute reported that some epidemiological studies also suggested that saccharin "is a weak carcinogen." The risk for humans, if it exists at all, is slight. The benefits of the sweetener, on the other hand, are both real and substantial. Saccharin is a boon to diabetics, who cannot use natural sugar. It is valuable in weight-reducing programs—and obesity is a proven risk factor for diabetes, high blood pressure and heart disease.

Perhaps the most moving of such controversies are over carcinogens that became well-nigh indispensable to modern ways of living before their dangers were detected. Sometimes even the victims of these killers ruefully ponder the dilemmas they pose. After many years of exposure to vinyl chloride in an Indiana factory manufacturing polyvinyl chloride plastic, Pete Gettelfinger came down with a rare cancer of the liver. The disease is almost always fatal; Pete died of it in 1975. Shortly before his death, he mused aloud to a visitor: "I think about this a lot—it's helped me a whole lot—the fact that we got 6,500 guys in the United States making a living working with polyvinyl chloride in the form I was using. If it wasn't for plastics, wood would be so expensive that the average man couldn't afford to have a rocking chair like this one where I'm sitting. And yet, it's killing people. It may kill me."

Five main types

For Pete Gettelfinger, the victim of a man-made carcinogen, the time for prevention had passed. But even if all man-made carcinogens were cleansed from the world, cancer cases would still occur, the disease arising from inescapable chemicals in the environment, induced by the rays of the sun or occurring spontaneously.

Most of these cancers can be avoided. Generally they can be cured. To plan a successful treatment, however, a physician must know the kind of cancer he is dealing with, the site of its origin and the extent of its spread. The most common type of cancer, called a carcinoma, grows in the linings of organs and in the skin. About one fifth as frequent and gener-

Subduing the terror of Lin Xian

A 20-square-mile corner of the Lin Xian valley in eastern China was a tragic pocket of cancer for at least 2,000 years. One in every four persons died of cancer of the esophagus, the tube leading to the stomach—a rate 250 times greater than the Chinese average. But, in one of the few instances in which a cancer cause has been unmistakably identified, Chinese scientists traced the disease to its origin and began to control the ancient terror of Lin Xian.

The program started in 1958 with attempts to isolate the cause. Local residents blamed the cancer on a habit of eating steaming-hot food. Food, it turned out, was involved, but not its temperature. The soil of Lin Xian is low in the element molybdenum. Without it, crops accumulate nitrite compounds; normally an enzyme containing molybdenum limits nitrites in living organisms.

The plants also produce less vitamin C, which helps eliminate nitrites. Hence the people of Lin Xian were building up high nitrite concentrations. At the same time, the foods they dried or pickled grew mold, considered a delicacy. The molds contain substances known as amines, which combine with nitrites to form nitrosamines. And nitrosamines cause esophageal cancer.

In early stages the cancer can be cured by surgery. In China trained technicians were assigned to screen residents of Lin Xian for treatment. And an educational campaign promoted preventive steps. It will be years before results can be gauged in lives saved, but villagers quickly began to treat fields with molybdenum and improve preserving techniques—measures to block the nitrosamines that had cursed Lin Xian with cancer.

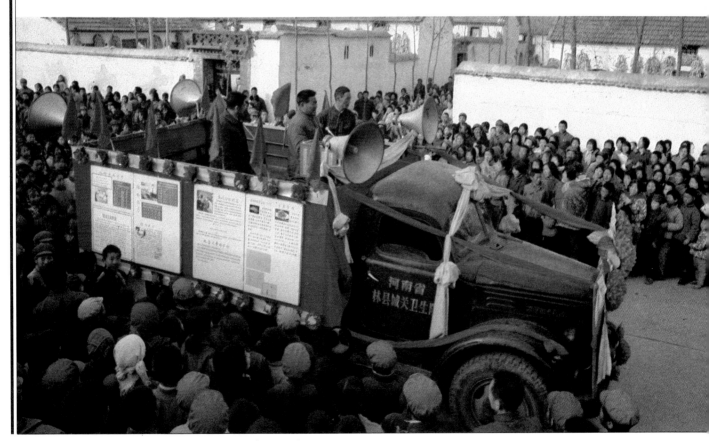

Its loudspeakers blaring a government message, a festooned truck draws a crowd in the campaign against the Lin Xian valley plague of esophageal cancer. Placards on the side of the truck describe the symptoms of the disease, name its causes and call upon the villagers to have medical checkups.

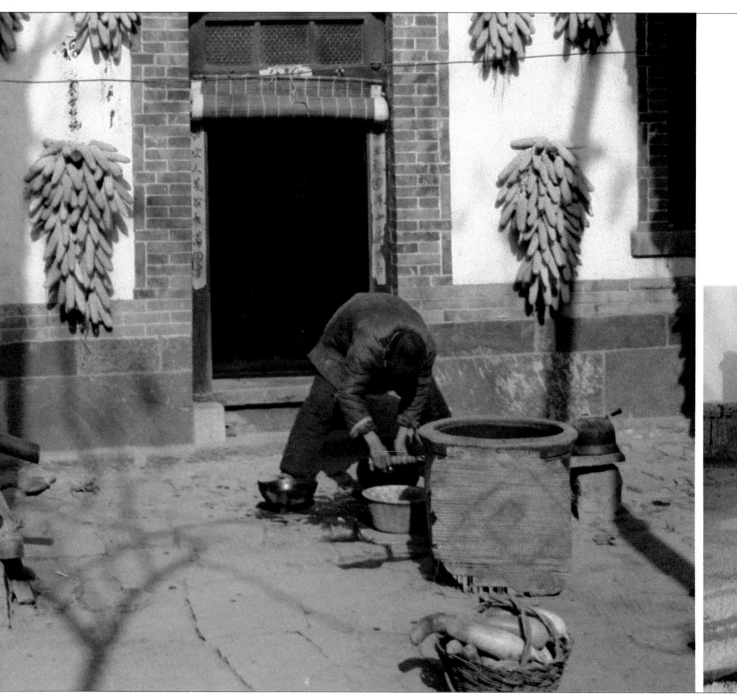

A Lin Xian peasant removes kernels from a corncob to preserve the food in a process that helps prevent cancer. When the corn was hung up to dry, as in the background, poor air circulation left enough moisture to produce cancer-inducing mold. Additional treatment (right) dries the kernels to prevent mold growth.

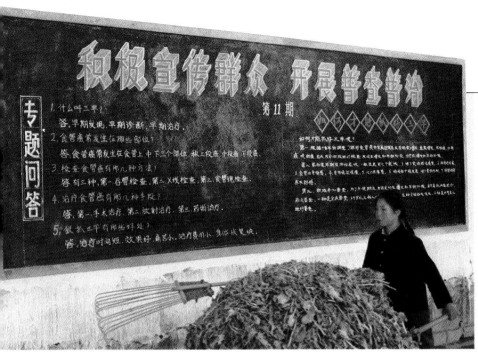

Her wheelbarrow laden with radishes, a young woman passes a billboard alerting villagers to ''the three earlies'' of cancer control: detection, diagnosis and treatment. Authorities also urge preservation of radishes and similar vegetables by proper drying rather than by pickling, which causes a mold blamed for cancer.

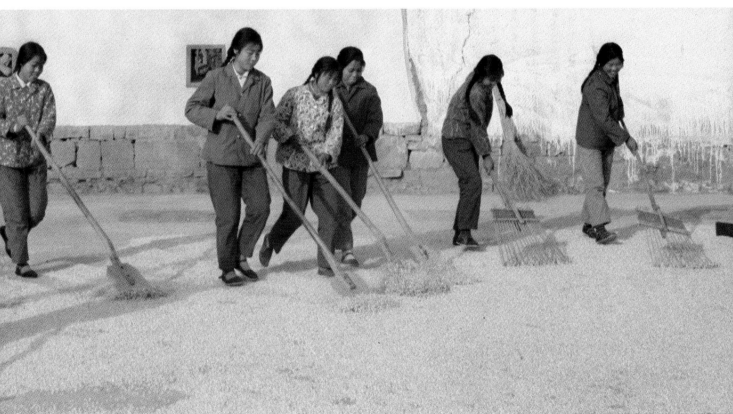

Wielding rakes and shovels, a team of young women spreads and turns piles of corn kernels to promote thorough drying. The technique they are using is part of the long-range campaign to eliminate mold from the diet of the people of Lin Xian and prevent the esophageal cancer that has plagued the region.

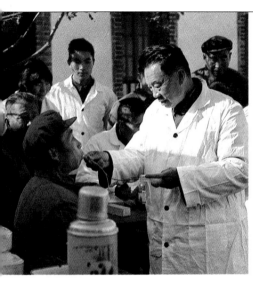

A technician administers the balloon test for esophageal cancer to a Lin Xian villager. The patient has swallowed a small balloon on the end of a rubber tube. When the balloon is then inflated and pulled out, it drags with it cells from the lining of the esophagus. Examination of these cells under a microscope reveals any malignancy.

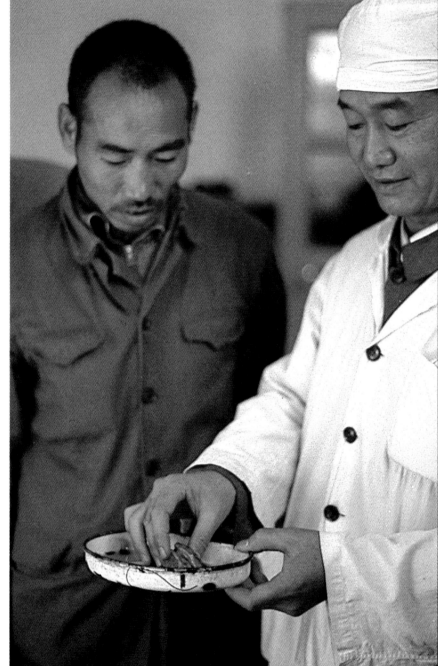

Moments after surgery, a doctor exhibits the esophageal tumors removed from this man's mother. Such visual demonstrations of the cancer's existence help impress on the people of Lin Xian the need for their cooperation in the war on the disease.

ally slower in growth are the sarcomas, found in bone, cartilage and muscle. Other major cancers include lymphomas, which, as their name implies, arise in the lymph system; myelomas, which start in the bone marrow; and leukemia, a cancer of blood-forming tissues.

Within these five divisions, cancer specialists distinguish more than 100 specific cancers, and further subdivisions easily double the number. Some are named for the organs they attack: A hepatoma, for example, is a cancer of the liver named from the Greek word *hepar,* or liver. Others bear the names of their discoverers: Wilms' tumor is named after Max Wilms, the German physician who studied it in 1899; the lymphoma called Hodgkin's disease bears the name of Thomas Hodgkin, the English pathologist who wrote the first accurate description of its symptoms in 1832.

Success in treating any type of cancer depends not only on identifying it but on identifying it early. Cancer cells spread widely, and the more they spread the more difficult they are to eradicate. Hodgkin's disease, for example, begins as a single mutant cell in a single node. The cell reproduces, splitting in half to form two cells. After about three years the growing mass of cells has doubled its number 20 times; it now contains about a million cells and weighs about $1/100$ gram—some 35/100,000 ounce. It is, of course, quite imperceptible at this stage, for it measures no more than 4/10,000 inch across. But at this point it has already sloughed off cells, perhaps hundreds or even thousands of them, and metastasized colonies may be growing elsewhere in the body. Not until the 30th doubling, when the original tumor contains about a billion cells, does it reach the size of a large pea. That pea-sized lump beneath the skin, perhaps in the abdomen or groin, is so subtle that many a victim has doubted his sense of touch.

The life-saving value of early detection and treatment is perhaps clearest in cases of lung cancer. The overall cure rate is a frightening 10 per cent—a one-in-10 chance of survival—because rarely can lung cancer be detected before it has spread to other parts of the body. If it is found before metastasis occurs, the survival rate leaps to 33 per cent.

One famous illustration of that fact is the case history of the radio and television personality Arthur Godfrey. In 1959 he consulted a physician about a persistent pain in his chest. An X-ray diagnosis was quick and clear: Godfrey's left lung contained a typical and common carcinoma, generally caused by smoking. The tumor had not metastasized, and the correct treatment was equally clear and straightforward: surgical removal. The operation was delicate—the tumor had grown around the aorta, the main artery from the heart—but it was successful. More than 20 years later Godfrey remained free of any sign of cancer.

Triumphs of treatment

The treatment of Arthur Godfrey's tumor was not only straightforward but classic. Since antiquity, the ideal way of curing cancer has been simply to cut it out. Ancient Greeks and Romans performed such operations, and in the 11th Century A.D., Abdul Qasim, an Arab physician practicing in Cordova, Spain, wrote a treatise on the state of his art that stands up well today. To begin with, he described situations that offer the best chance of cure: "When a cancer is in a site where total eradication is possible, such as a cancer of the breast or of the thigh, and in similar parts where complete removal is possible, and especially when in the early stage and small, then surgery is to be tried." Modern surgical techniques have greatly expanded the list of possible sites for surgery; today, cancers such as those of the lung and liver, which were considered inoperable as recently as the 1950s, are removed almost as effectively as the superficial tumors of skin cancer.

Abdul Qasim also recognized the limitations of the scalpel. "When the cancer is of long standing and large," he wrote, "you should leave it alone. For I myself have never been able to cure any such, nor have I seen anyone else succeed before me." Size and age of the tumor are only two of the considerations that can make surgery impractical. If a tumor has engulfed a vital organ or grown far into adjacent tissues, the damage done by the knife may be as devastating as that of the cancer itself. Tiny metastases scattered throughout the body are generally impervious to surgery, and some systemic cancers, such as those of the blood or the lymphatic system, offer no possible site for an operation.

When surgery is impossible or ill-advised, the cancer fighter turns to newer weapons in his arsenal. One is radiation therapy, in which, as in a science-fiction story, death-dealing rays are brought to bear on an alien invader. Another is chemotherapy, the science of poisoning cancer cells with drugs. Both are products of the 20th Century and are still undergoing rapid development, but both have become standard tools in the battle against cancer.

Often prescribed for solid tumors that are inoperable because of their size or location, radiation almost always stops the growth of cancer and sometimes shrinks it enough to make surgery possible. In principle, the treatment is simple. The rays focused upon a tumor may be powerful X-rays, or the emanations of a radioactive element, or the subatomic particles produced in an atom smasher. Any cell that is in the process of reproduction is disrupted by the rays, but cancer cells, which repair themselves less well than healthy ones, are more likely to be destroyed. To improve the odds still further, elaborate shields protect the healthy cells from lethal rays *(pages 110-121)* and sometimes radioactive pellets are delivered directly to the heart of a tumor on wires or in needles.

Chemotherapy is the newest treatment of all—productive work in the field did not begin until the 1950s. It is also the most miraculously effective. It is, in fact, responsible for most of the victories against cancer in recent years, because it attacks types of systemic cancer once beyond the reach of any treatment. Hodgkin's disease and leukemia, for example, are generally widespread before they are detected, but drugs introduced into the bloodstream will attack them everywhere in the body. Similarly, the most minute metastases are vulnerable to chemotherapy. A physician need not know the precise locations of these pockets of danger; the drugs will seek them out.

The cancer fighter generally deploys more than one kind of weapon; a combination suited to specific cancers and patients is more effective. Surgery or radiation of an original tumor may be backed up by chemotherapy to eliminate metastases, and as many as 10 drugs may be used in combination or succession to kill every last malignant cell. Or any of the three therapies may begin a course of treatment to reduce the size of a large tumor, with the others coming in as needed.

Each of the three brings its own risks and costs. Surgery is never completely safe, and cancer surgery can be disfiguring. Radiation and chemotherapy can be hazardous even when closely monitored, and both have side effects ranging from mild discomfort to outright illness. But for many patients the very harshness of cancer treatments comes as a challenge to fight the disease through. Ruth Cullen, a victim of Hodgkin's disease, noticed that her first dose of anti-cancer drugs came in a syringe labeled POISON. "It was a turning point," she recalled. "It marked a real loss of innocence. Up until then, I hadn't admitted that there was anything wrong inside. Putting that stuff in there made it very real to me that there was something inside my body that was trying to kill me." Two years later, after a grueling course of radiation and chemotherapy, not a trace of her disease could be found—and she felt, she said, "like one of a charmed circle."

The worldwide army of cancer fighters

To enter that circle, a cancer patient must get the right treatment, in the right amount, at the right time. Not all do. Dr. Juan del Regato of the University of South Florida, in a comprehensive textbook on cancer treatment, wryly described various hurdles on the path to the best possible treatment. They include, he wrote, "wishful thinking (to which physicians are not immune), geography, luck, misinformation (lay and professional), organization, luck, facilities, skills and a great deal of luck."

The hurdles are real enough, yet almost every cancer victim can leap over all of them—including the hurdle of luck. A worldwide network of laboratories and hospitals, of research scientists and physicians, has been established to pursue the search for cancer cures, exchange information on new findings and therapies, and make the best professional services available to every patient who needs them.

If any single event can be said to have started this network, it would be the passage of the National Cancer Act by the

United States Congress in 1971. The Act appropriated funds for cancer research; more important, it empowered the National Cancer Institute to coordinate research and treatment programs and to give support to investigators and physicians throughout the nation and the world. By 1975, in the United States alone, 670,000 people were at work on the problems of cancer's cause and cure. In 1971 the Institute spent $230 million; within a decade its annual budget rose to one billion dollars.

Though instigated and largely financed by the United States, the war against cancer is directed and fought internationally. The European Organization for Research on Treatment of Cancer coordinates experiments at more than 80 cancer centers spread across Europe, from Portugal to Germany and from Norway to Sicily. Elsewhere, the work is coordinated through national cancer research centers in Japan, China and the Soviet Union. And information from all these sources is regularly exchanged—much of it over a globe-girdling computer network—for the benefit of researchers, physicians and patients everywhere.

This immense effort has already paid for itself in new knowledge of cancer, new treatments and—best of all—enormous advances in survival and cure rates. Most of the work on cancer prevention has been directly or indirectly supported by the organized network of cancer researchers; and the ongoing, sometimes tedious work of sifting laboratory findings would be inconceivable without it. Chemotherapy, for example, is a young science, but one that depends mainly upon large-scale tests and trials rather than the inspired work of individual geniuses. Over a quarter century, some 700,000 natural and synthetic chemotherapeutic drugs were screened. Of this number, only 50 proved useful and became commercially available.

For the cancer patient, the effort has paid off in new facilities, new medical equipment and sophisticated treatment. To a great degree, the hurdles described by Dr. del Regato—geography, organization, skill and the rest—are down. Worldwide, 680 research and treatment institutions in 82 countries serve the potential or actual cancer victim. In the United States, more than 90 per cent of the population lives within 200 miles of one of the institutions described by the National Cancer Institute as cancer centers, which offer the most up-to-date cancer treatment and also carry on research into new methods of treatment. And in any hospital specializing in cancer care, a patient can expect certain standardized, effective modes of diagnosis and treatment.

The rigor and thoroughness of these modes can be seen in the sequence of steps, called a protocol, in the treatment of cancer of the colon, or lower intestine. To begin with, a doctor takes a look at the interior of the colon, using an instrument called a sigmoidoscope or colonoscope. If he finds a tumorous growth, he calls upon specialists to perform a biopsy—to remove a piece of it for laboratory analysis to determine whether it is benign or malignant. Usually, he will want the growth cut out in either case.

If the growth is a polyp, or small tumor, and is located near the rectum, the doctor himself may remove it. To treat a growth further up the colon, he will call in a surgeon, who also proceeds according to the steps of a protocol. The surgeon generally removes a benign tumor by simply cutting it away at its base; when operating on a malignant tumor, he removes a portion of the colon above and below the growth as well. If the portion is relatively small, the severed ends of the colon are sewed together; if it is large, an opening is made in the wall of the abdomen to let the patient pass bowel movements into a plastic pouch. Finally, to complete the protocol, surgery is generally followed by chemotherapy or by a combination of radiation therapy and chemotherapy.

Such treatments are the work of skilled scientists and craftsmen—the professional soldiers in the war against cancer. The ranks of such professionals range from the field marshals who direct the national and international campaigns, down to the foot soldiers who run tests in laboratories. By comparison, the potential cancer victim is a civilian, who may seem helpless while the battle rages. But this civilian can prevent the battle by simply avoiding the disease. A handful of common cancer-causing agents is responsible for most of the cancer in the world. Armed with knowledge and prudence, the civilians in the cancer war have it in their power to deny cancer most of its chances to attack. ✸

Eleven-month-old Jamie Russ, her leukemia detected a month earlier, toddles across Oncology Street's playroom, supervised by her father, Robert. The red mark on the girl's cheek—indelible ink—helps target the X-rays used in her treatment.

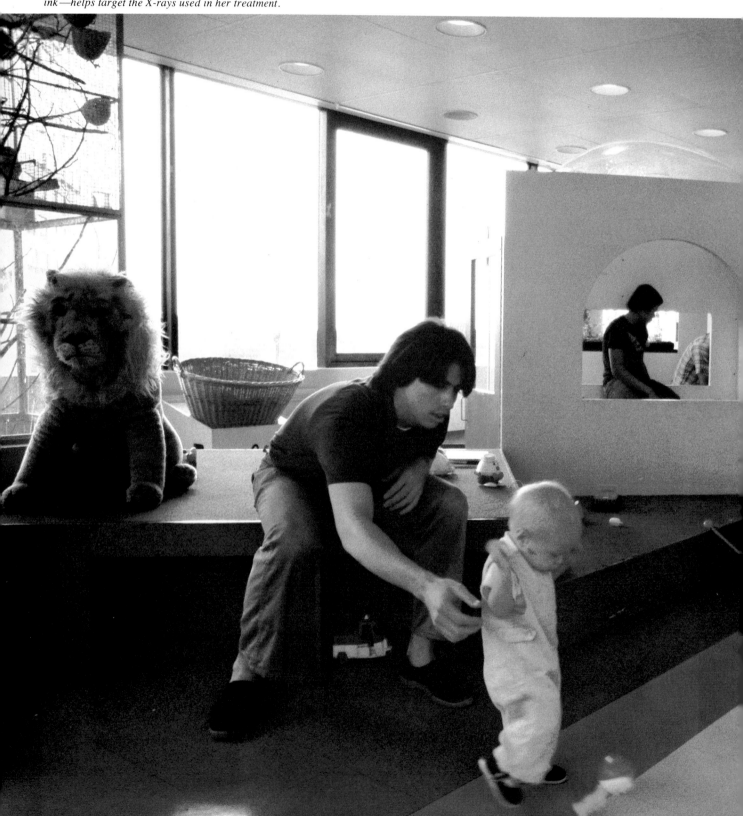

A special place for saving children

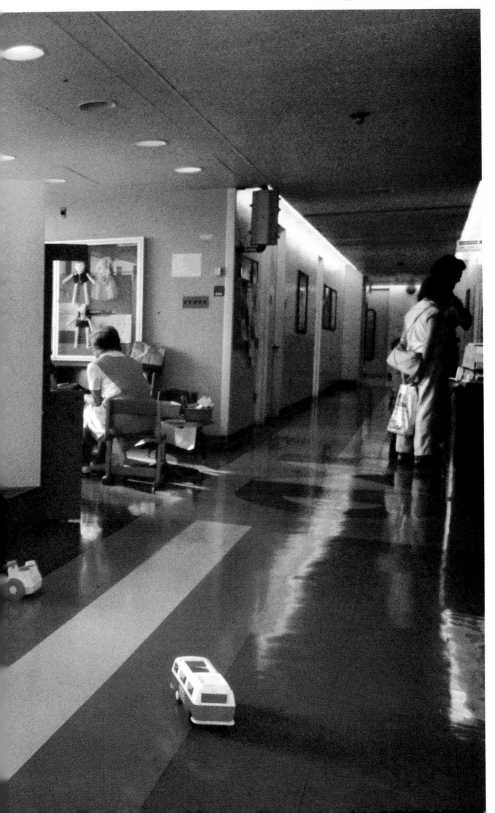

"Oncology Street," announces the small red sign in the hallway leading to the cancer clinic at The Children's Hospital of Philadelphia. From the moment a young cancer patient sees the street, he senses this is no ordinary doctor's office. The spacious, sunny playroom *(left)* at the entrance to Oncology Street is filled with toys, games and other diversions, including a 40-gallon aquarium and a floor-to-ceiling cage populated by noisy finches.

Indeed, Oncology Street is a special place, not only a clinic where childhood cancers, mainly leukemia, are studied, treated—and often cured—but also a place where patients and their families are made to feel at home.

Oncology Street's cheerful, homey atmosphere is carefully calculated. Especially for children, physical health and emotional well-being go hand in hand. For physical health, the clinic employs advanced therapies to fight leukemia, a cancer of the blood-forming tissues—in the bone marrow, the spleen and the lymph glands. For emotions, the environment brims with love and optimism.

The love is natural, the optimism justified. Since the 1950s, medical science has transformed leukemia from an almost uniformly fatal affliction to a curable disease. New drugs can kill the malignant blood cells, and modern supportive therapies—transfusions, antibiotics and high-protein intravenous feedings—can give badly weakened patients time to recover. As a result, more than 50 per cent of the children with the most common variant of the disease, acute lymphocytic leukemia, survive at least five years past diagnosis.

"Ten years ago," said Dr. Audrey E. Evans, Director of Oncology at Children's Hospital and the driving force behind Oncology Street, "we were hesitant even to use the word 'cure.' We now can confidently say that we cure more than half the patients we see."

The benefits flowing from this combination of professional skill and loving care are not lost on the patients. Said one 13-year-old, "It's fun to go. I don't think about the treatment. I think about talking to everyone."

PHOTOGRAPHS BY LINDA BARTLETT

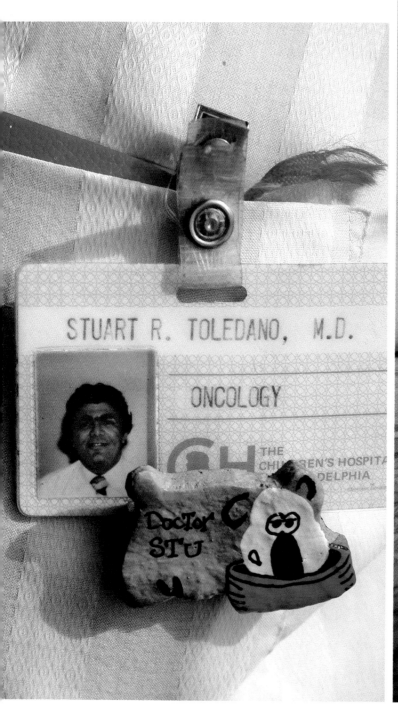

Dr. Stu, a papier-mâché puppy, enlivens
the badge of Dr. Stuart R. Toledano.
He added the ornament partly to distract the
young patients and partly "because none
of them can pronounce my name."

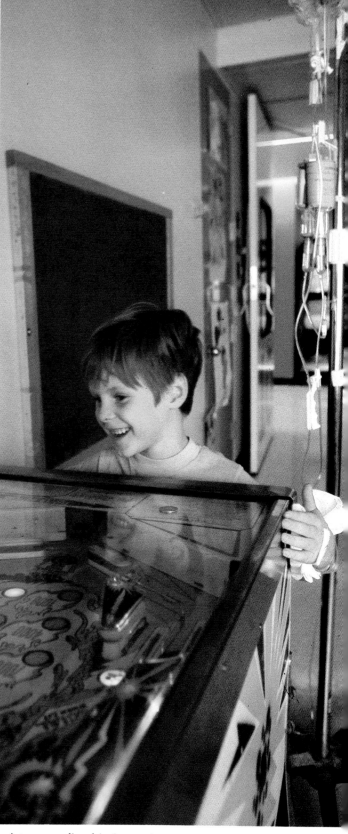

An intravenous line dripping nutrients
into a vein in his arm, six-year-old Derek
Steinmetz delights in his success at a
pinball game. The machine was a gift from
the parents of a patient.

Two young cancer sufferers—Bobby Lake, aged three, and Richard Ruch, aged five—try their hand at artwork. Helping them is Carol Vermeil, one of a staff of eight volunteer play therapists.

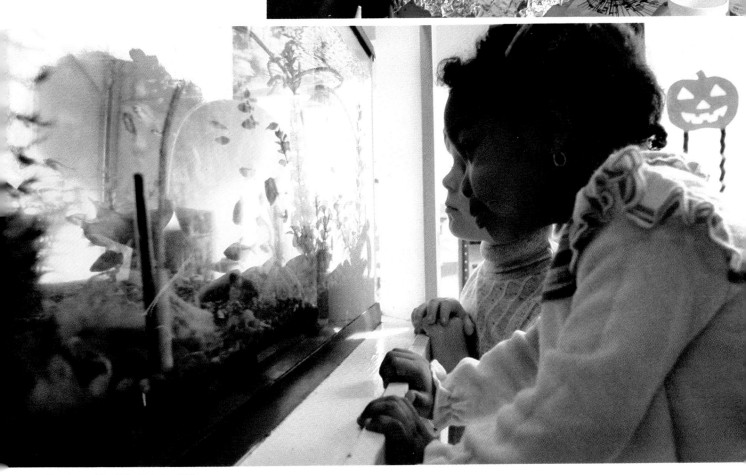

Fascinated by fish, Kristina Wilson passes time before her treatment by observing Oncology Street's aquarium. Another gift from a patient's parents, it is one of the playroom's most popular attractions.

Keeping tabs on the patient's progress

It is only a few short steps from the fun and games of Oncology Street's playroom to the serious and sometimes scary business of the medical areas. Treatments vary, but all include repeated physical examinations.

Many tests are routine probings—weight and height measurements, blood pressure checks, blood sampling. For a child suffering from leukemia, however, even standard examinations assume a special significance. Changes in blood pressure, body temperature or weight may warn of side effects from anti-leukemia drugs. Routine blood samples can indicate a drug's effectiveness.

Some examinations are not routine, for complex tests are needed to track spreading cancerous cells. Unlike most normal blood cells, leukemia cells easily cross the so-called blood-brain barrier and infiltrate the liquid that cushions the brain and spinal cord. To find out if malignant cells are lurking there, the doctors must obtain some of the fluid. The only way to do that is by a painful and understandably unpopular spinal tap.

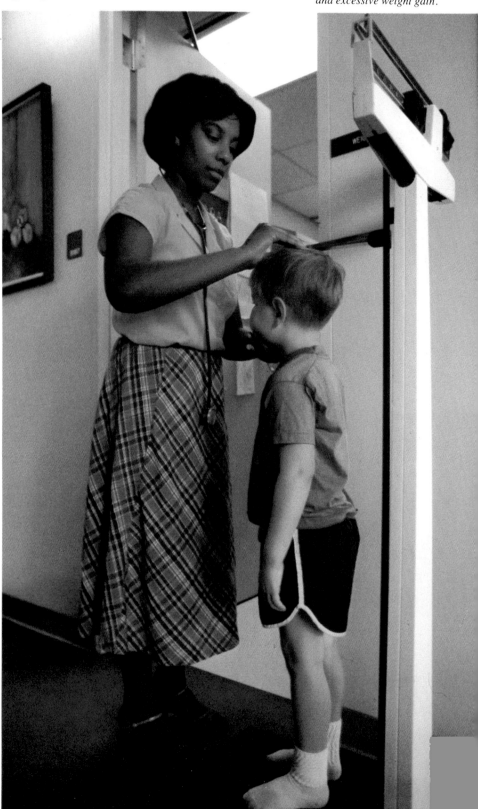

Richard Ruch stretches tall while his height and weight are checked. During his three years of treatment for leukemia, Richard received prednisone, a drug that can lead to both high blood pressure and excessive weight gain.

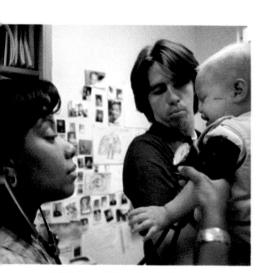

Held by her father, Jamie Russ cries as her blood pressure is measured to check the effect of a drug she was receiving.

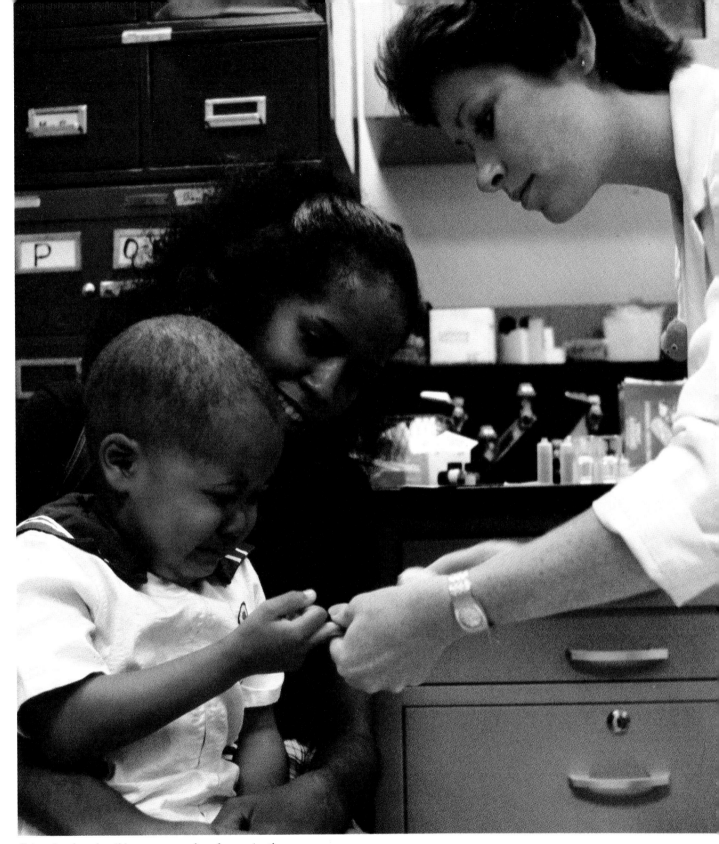

Grimacing from bewilderment as much as from pain, three-year-old Philip Downing has his finger pricked for a blood test. Blood is dripped into a glass cylinder, then spun in a centrifuge, which, like a cream separator pulling cream out of milk, separates blood cells for a check of drugs' effects on them.

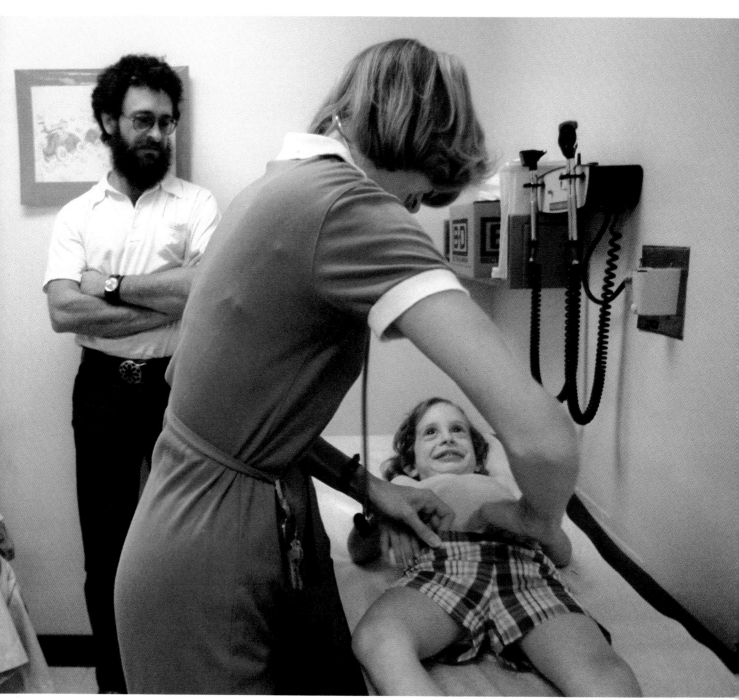

Grinning four-year-old Matthew Elliott, stricken by leukemia at the age of two, endures a slightly ticklish examination by Dr. Rebecca L. Byrd, as his father looks on. Dr. Byrd is feeling Matthew's spleen and liver, organs often infiltrated by leukemia cells. If these organs are swollen, malignant cells probably are present. That day, Matthew's spleen and liver felt normal.

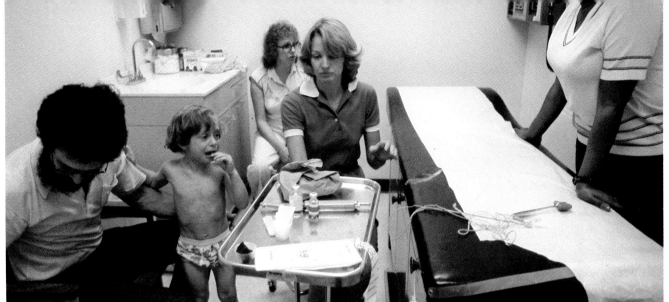

His smile gone, Matthew breaks into tears at a familiar and menacing sight—the cart that holds the implements used to tap fluid around the spine. Analysis of the fluid reveals if cancer has spread there.

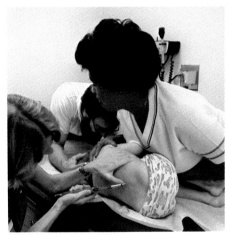

Matthew's father and a nurse's aide hold the boy as Dr. Byrd numbs his skin with anesthetic before she inserts the large spinal needle—about as thick as a pencil lead—between the vertebrae.

Protruding from Matthew's spinal cavity, a needle drips spinal fluid into a test tube. The fluid was clear, not cloudy, indicating it was free of cancer cells, a welcome result confirmed later by laboratory analysis.

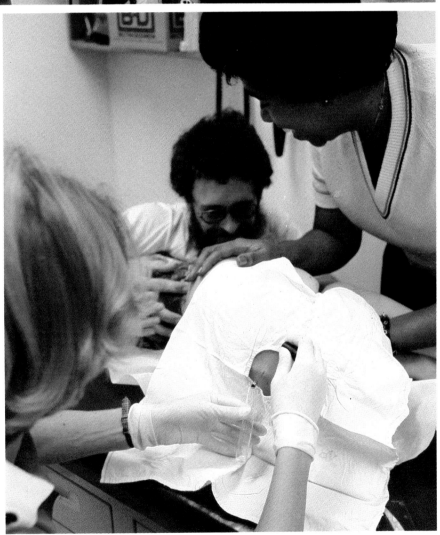

The tricky business of treating leukemia

Leukemia is a notoriously resilient disease. It can be present in full force one week, then, stunned by drugs, it may be impossible to detect and seemingly defeated the next. Yet it can reappear weeks or years later, as dangerous as ever. Thus doctors first try to eliminate all signs of the disease—produce a remission. Then they fight to extend the remission so that the temporary interlude is stretched on and on into a cure.

In the first stage of the attack, called induction, leukemia is blitzed by powerful combinations of drugs, some of which can produce unpleasant side effects. For the most common form of leukemia, acute lymphocytic leukemia, abbreviated ALL, three drugs are generally given: vincristine, to keep leukemia cells from dividing; l-asparaginase, to block protein production and starve the cells; and prednisone, to kill cells directly.

To kill the malignant cells that might be lurking around the brain and spinal cord, cancer-killing radiation and another drug that stops cell reproduction—usually methotrexate—are used. Such treatments bring remission to nearly 95 per cent of the patients with ALL, often within two weeks. Their symptoms disappear, and they feel fine.

But to stay in remission, a patient must come to the clinic periodically for additional treatments, many the same as those used for induction. Unlike the brief induction treatment, however, maintenance therapy normally lasts two to three years.

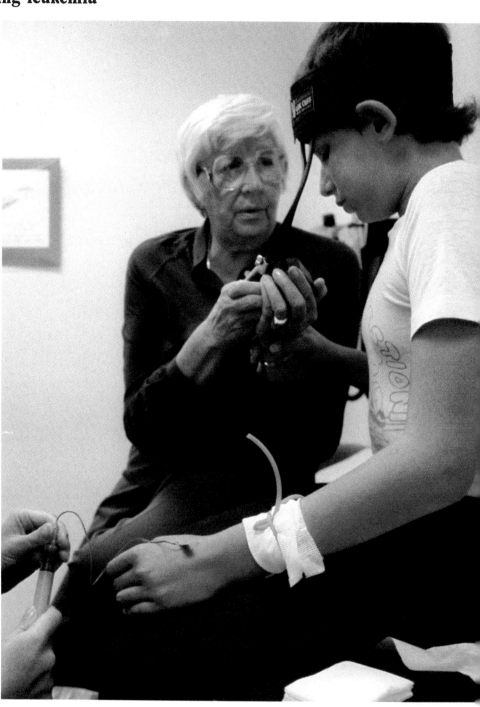

An inflatable head tourniquet protects 13-year-old Danny Peshkin from one effect of vincristine, the drug he is receiving. The tourniquet, operated by his grandmother, reduces circulation in his scalp to keep the drug from reaching his hair follicles; vincristine can harm them, causing hair loss.

Asleep with her stuffed elephant, Bimbo, Stephanie Arndt, 17, receives intravenous fluid through a tube attached to her hand. Minutes earlier, the tube carried cyclophosphamide, an anticancer drug; the follow-up fluid, a salt-sugar solution, is to counteract dehydration if the drug causes vomiting.

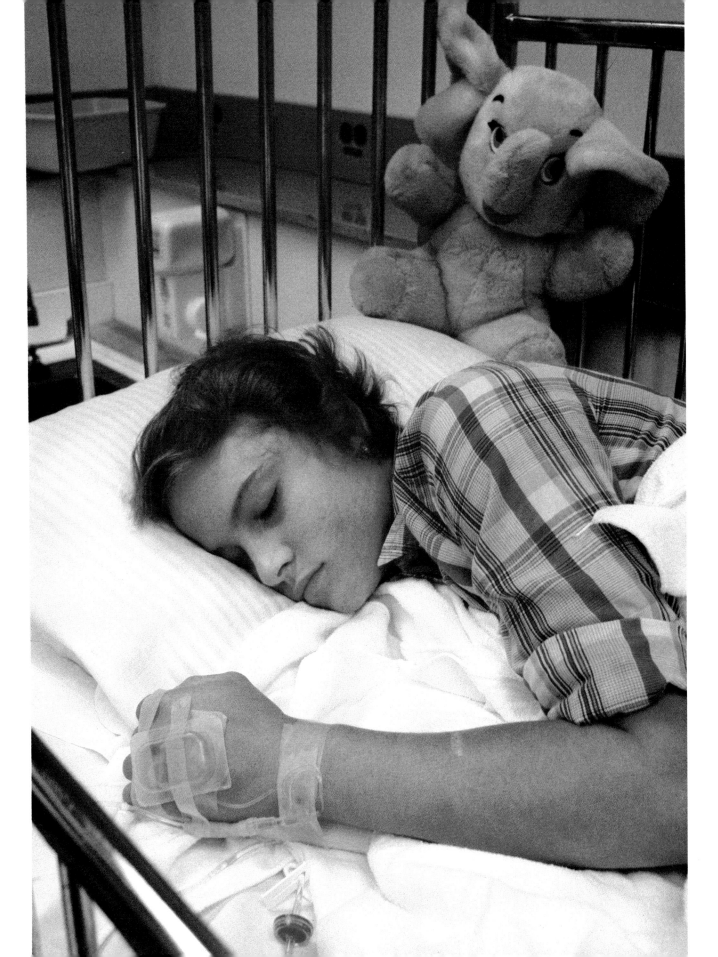

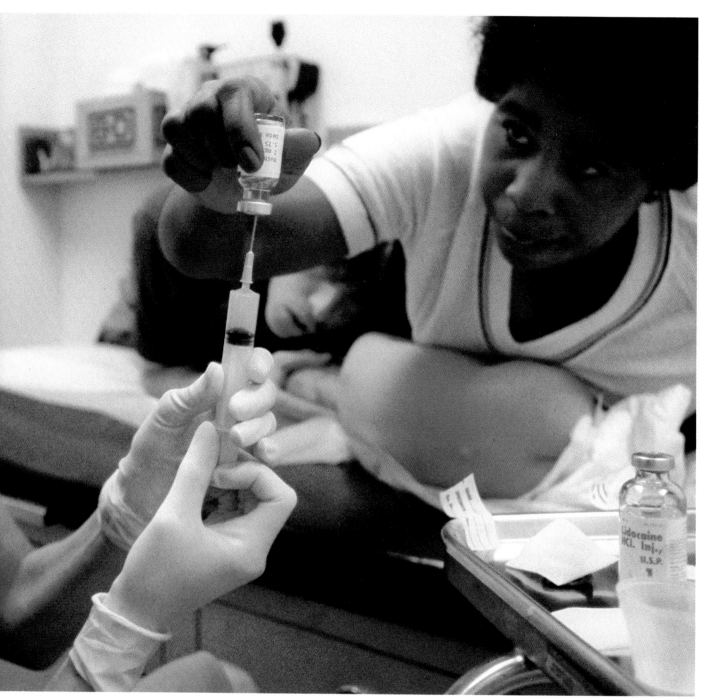

A syringe is filled with the drug methotrexate for a spinal injection. A patient with the common leukemia known as ALL normally receives six such injections during the first two months of treatment; after that, methotrexate may be administered every three months for as long as three years.

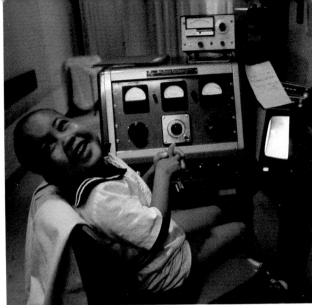

As delighted as if he were the captain
of his own spaceship, Philip Downing hams
it up (left) at the controls of an X-
ray machine. Below, his head is taped to
the treatment table to keep the cancer
target steady in the X-ray beam. A nurse
uses a ruler to check that the distance
from the machine is correct. During this
procedure, a beam of light simulates
the X-ray beam that will kill leukemia cells.

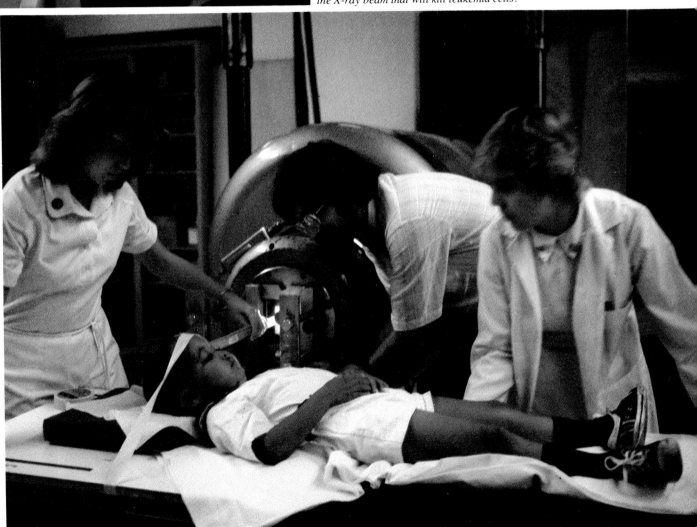

In-patient care: home away from home

Although most treatments can be completed during a few hours' visit to the Children's Hospital clinic, all patients must stay over for at least a few days and nights. For some patients, that is the only time they spend the night in the hospital, and usually a parent sleeps in a cot alongside. But for a child who must undergo special treatments, longer and more frequent stays are necessary.

One operation requiring long-term hospitalization is a bone-marrow transplant, which replaces cancerous blood-forming tissue with healthy tissue from someone else. This procedure is complicated by the fact that the white blood cells produced by bone marrow—the ones involved in leukemia—are the same ones that protect the body against foreign invaders, such as disease germs. Unless the donated marrow is similar to the replaced marrow in its genetic character, that is, in its heredity-controlling DNA molecules, it will produce blood cells that attack the recipient's tissues, believing them to be foreign.

For this reason, the donor must be someone who shares the same heredity as the recipient—a very close relative. An identical twin is best, a brother or sister next best, and a parent somewhat less satisfactory.

The role of bone marrow in fighting disease adds yet another complication. Because the patient's own marrow has been replaced, and because the transplanted marrow takes time to regain normal strength, the recipient is temporarily virtually defenseless against infection. For protection, he must stay in a sterile isolation room, sometimes for three months.

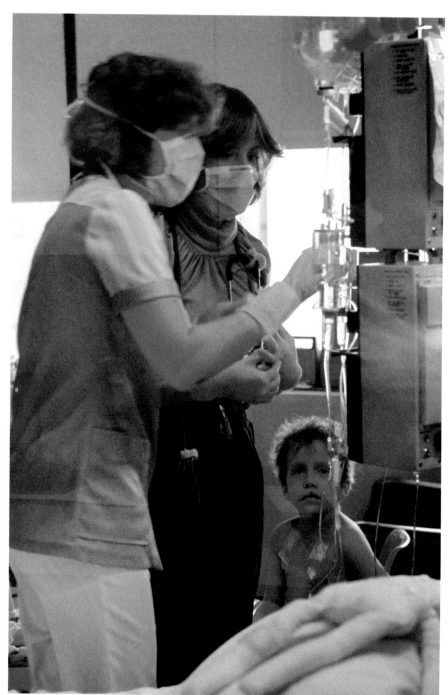

Five days after a bone-marrow transplant, Kirk Horvath—seen through reflections in the window of his isolation room—looks on while two nurses adjust tubes that drip nutrients into his body. The nurses wear masks and gloves to prevent infecting the six-year-old, whose treatment has nullified his disease defenses.

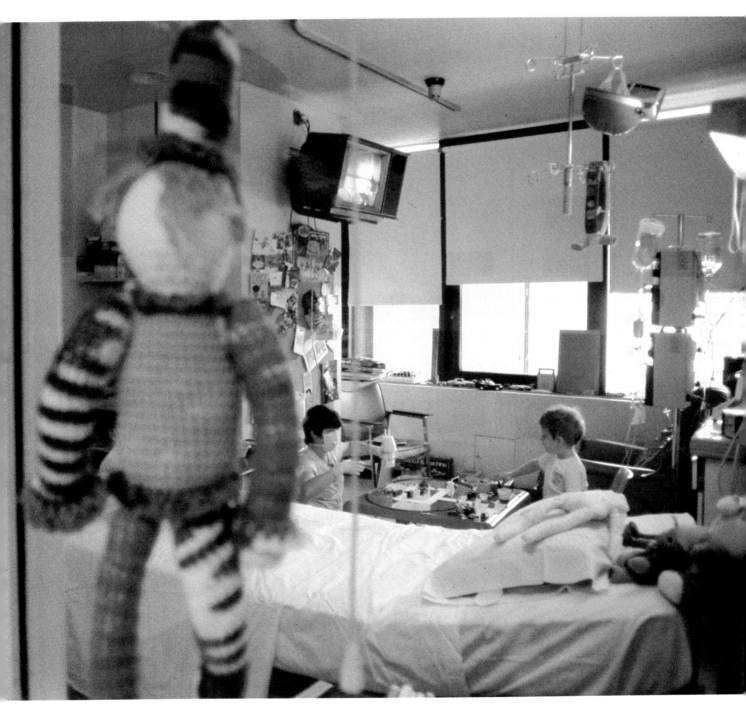

A stuffed clown and other mementos from home soften the impact of Kirk's hospital stay; so does the presence of his mother, who must wear mask and gloves while entertaining him. Mrs. Horvath donated bone marrow to save her son. Seven weeks later, Kirk was home, past a major hurdle on the road to recovery.

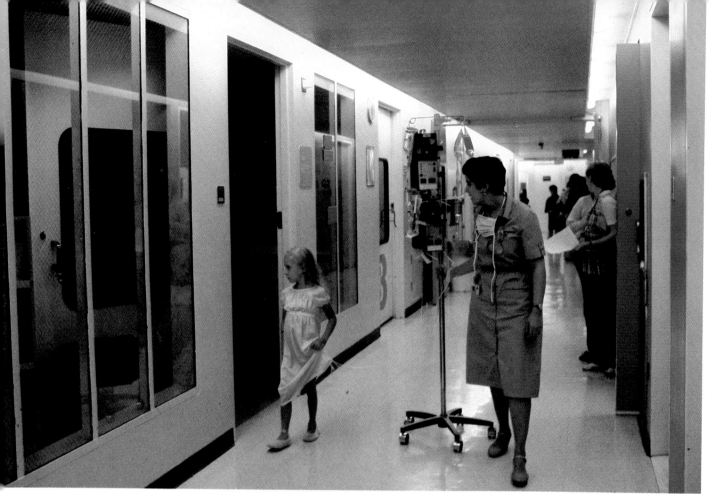

Heather Gondolf, aged six, strolls a hospital corridor while a nurse maneuvers a wheeled pole holding the intravenous supplies to which Heather is attached.

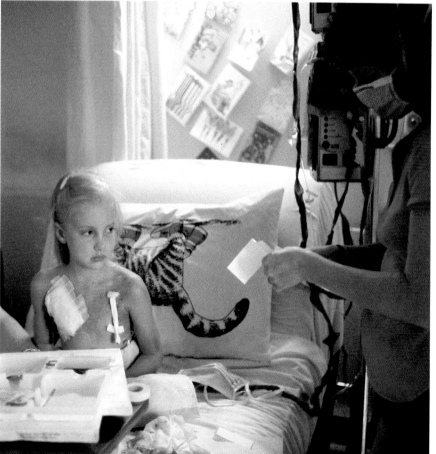

Seated in her hospital bed, Heather watches intently while a nurse prepares to change the dressing on one of her intravenous lines. The tubes carry high-calorie liquid nourishment, antileukemia drugs and antibiotics to treat an infection.

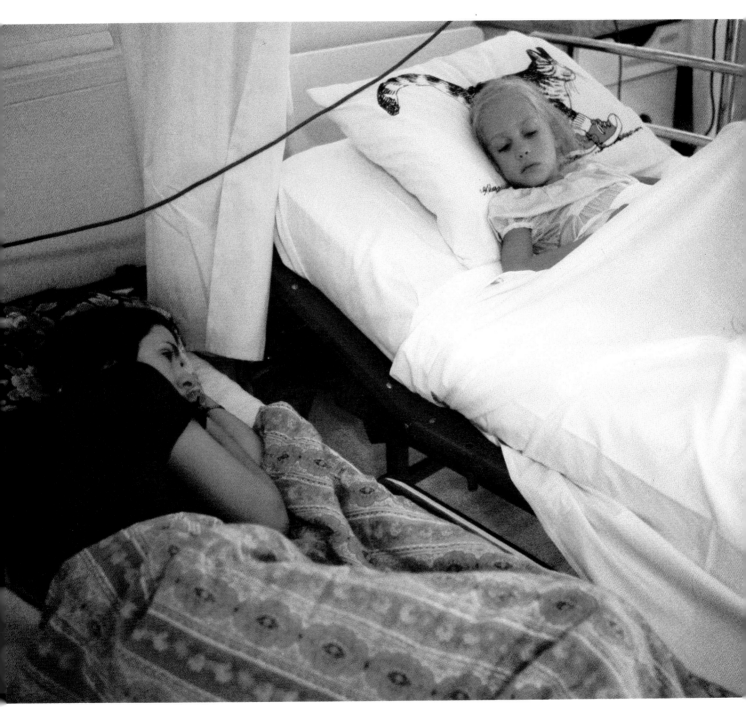

On a cot next to her daughter, Mrs. Gondolf watches Heather sleep in the morning light. Unless a child is in isolation, parents are encouraged to stay in their child's room overnight. If a whole family must come from out of town, a nearby town house, bought with a donation, provides low-cost accommodations.

A decade of progress on Oncology Street

When Oncology Street opened in 1970, said its director, Dr. Evans, "20 to 30 per cent of the cancer patients we were seeing were being cured." The figure rose steadily. By the mid-1970s it stood at nearly 45 per cent. And after a decade, the doctors of Oncology Street could predict cure for about 60 per cent of the approximately 250 new patients they see each year.

Such remarkable lifesaving is not unique to Children's Hospital—the victory over childhood malignancies is the outstanding success story of cancer treatment—but the Philadelphia institution is one of the select few around the world that have led the way in these advances. It is the headquarters, for example, for a nationwide study of Wilms' tumor, a relatively rare cancer of the kidney. Partly as a result of the Children's Hospital efforts, the cure rate for Wilms' tumor rose during Oncology Street's first decade from near 50 per cent to almost 90 per cent.

These successes charge the atmosphere of Oncology Street. Gay colors, toys and pets *(right)* are more than a psychological boost for severely ill youngsters; they are symbols of solid optimism. Children with cancer now have a future that may soon be as bright and long and normal as that of children who have never had the disease.

Seven-year-old Stacy Thompson accepts
from Dr. Audrey E. Evans, Director
of Oncology at Children's Hospital, two of
Oncology Street's white finches—the
standard gift to a young patient going home.

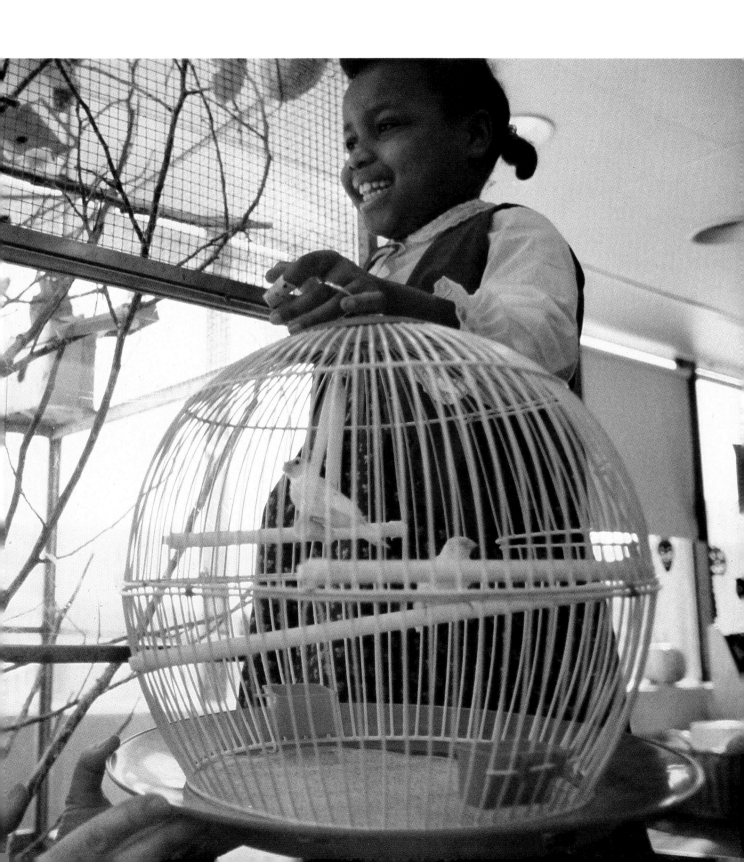

CHAPTER 2

Sidestepping the causes

The facts about cigarettes
How to stop smoking for good
Food: cause and preventive
Perilous additives
Why to avoid a fashionable tan
The occupational hazards

Like most smokers, Linda and her husband, Arnold, had tried repeatedly to stop. Like many, they had failed each time. Then, while getting over a bad cold, Linda developed a cough that would not go away. Alarmed, she and Arnold made a pact to give up cigarettes totally and at once.

''I was depressed for months,'' Linda recalled, ''and Arnold was so crabby you had to measure every word before speaking to him. But we stuck to our decision. Neither of us has had one cigarette since we agreed to stop, and that was 15 years ago.''

No one can know whether Linda's cough was a warning of an oncoming cancer. But the couple was well aware of the link between smoking and lung cancer and knew that the cough could have been a signal. Possibly, their decision to stop smoking prevented them from contracting lung cancer and perhaps saved their lives.

Such thoughts, reported by Jane Brody in her book *You Can Fight Cancer and Win,* are entertained by countless other former smokers who have kicked the habit in the decades since the incriminating evidence against smoking became widely known. Giving up tobacco is not the only thing a person can do to prevent cancer, and not even the only measure that can be taken to avoid lung cancer. Other substances, agents and habits have been associated with both lung cancer and a host of other forms of the disease. Thus avoiding the ''things'' that cause cancer—carcinogens—can reduce dramatically the risk of falling prey to the disease. Doctors are convinced, in fact, that fully one quarter of the

life-threatening cancers that occur each year could be prevented if people would make certain significant but easily managed changes in the way they live.

The idea that much cancer is preventable arises from research in the years after World War II. Until then the prevailing belief was that cancer was largely hereditary. Indeed, there is considerable evidence to suggest that genetic traits may make one family more cancer prone than another. Women whose mothers, sisters or aunts have had breast cancer, for example, are twice as likely to develop the disease as those whose relatives have not been afflicted. But so much has been learned about outside influences that can bring on malignancies that environmental factors now are universally accepted as producing 70 to 90 per cent of all cancers.

''From what you hear,'' said one New York woman, echoing a widespread belief, ''everything these days causes cancer.'' Sunlight, coffee, X-rays, and chemicals such as benzene and arsenic have been implicated. Indeed, as a member of modern technological society, you are living in a sea of carcinogens. They are in the air you breathe, the food you eat, the drugs you take and even the clothing you wear. They can be influenced by where and how you live, by what you do for a living, and by your idiosyncracies and habits.

But, as cancer producers, they are not all created equal. Some are far more dangerous than others, and some that generate the biggest headlines are among the least dangerous. What is more, many of the most dangerous carcinogens—tobacco, for instance—are almost entirely avoid-

A dramatic poster drives home a sobering fact: Cigarettes can be as lethal as a loaded gun. Masses of evidence from decades of statistical and laboratory research demonstrate that smoking increases the risk of lung cancer as much as 20 times.

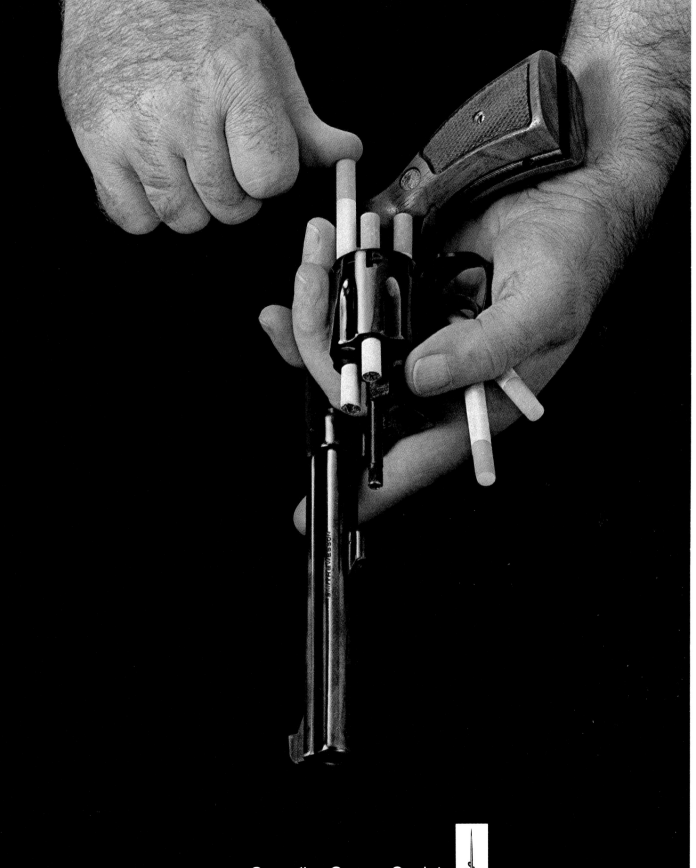

Canadian Cancer Society

able. A host of others are at least partially avoidable, so that exposure to them can be minimized.

When the causes are ones over which you have little or no control, such as heredity, the best protection is vigilance. Learn about changes in the body that can signal the presence of cancer, and perform religiously the self-examinations that can reveal it at an early stage. At the first hint that something might be wrong, see a doctor: The sooner a physician can begin treatment, the greater the likelihood that the threat will be contained.

The facts about cigarettes

Of all the cancer threats in the sea of carcinogens, perhaps the worst—but certainly the one most readily blocked—is the common cigarette. In Westernized countries smoking is the principal cause of more than one fourth of all cancer deaths among men and of a growing percentage among women. Lung cancer—mostly derived from cigarette smoking—is almost alone in bringing about the 50 per cent increase in the overall United States cancer death rate during the past generation. In that time, lung-cancer death rates have risen more than 2,500 per cent, while death rates for other forms of the disease have either declined or risen only slightly.

The rise in lung cancer throughout the world can be tied directly to cigarettes. Early in the 20th Century, when cigarette smoking first was gaining acceptance among men, lung cancer was almost unheard-of. Medical records of 1912, for example, reveal a mere 374 cases of lung cancer for the entire world. About that time, however, a new, milder type of tobacco was developed in Virginia. It could be inhaled deep into the lungs without inducing coughing fits and a choking sensation. Between 1910 and 1920, the average yearly consumption of cigarettes in the United States rose from around four billion to almost 25 billion.

Almost immediately suspicions were aroused, because the boom in cigarette consumption paralleled an increase in deaths from lung cancer. In 1921 Dr. Moses Barron of the University of Minnesota reported that in the two decades between 1899 and 1918, only four cases of death from lung cancer had been found in nearly 4,000 autopsies at the uni-

versity. In just two years, between 1919 and 1921, by contrast, there were nine lung-cancer deaths in 1,033 autopsies—an 800 per cent increase.

Subsequent research was slow to confirm Dr. Barron's findings. Scientists years later would be able to say why: Lung cancer takes 20 or more years to develop; it has what doctors call a long latency period. The big rise in lung cancer would not begin to show until the 1940s and 1950s.

Meantime, cigarette consumption boomed. As the number of smokers mounted, so did evidence from around the world of tobacco's lethal effects. In the United States an enterprising medical student named Ernst Wynder persuaded one of his professors at Washington University in St. Louis, Dr. Evarts Graham, to investigate the relationship between rising lung-cancer deaths and the growing popularity of cigarettes. Dr. Graham, a heavy smoker (as were approximately 60 per cent of American physicians at the time), was skeptical. But in 1949 they studied the records of 684 lung-cancer patients at Washington University's hospital. They found that 94 per cent of the patients were cigarette smokers and that most of the remainder smoked either pipes or cigars; fewer than 2 per cent had never smoked. Among patients who did not have lung cancer, almost 15 per cent were nonsmokers.

In the May 1950 *Journal of the American Medical Association,* Dr. Graham and Wynder stated: ''Extensive and prolonged use of tobacco, especially cigarettes, seems to be an important factor in the inducement of bronchogenic carcinoma.'' (For his part, Dr. Graham swore off cigarettes, but it was too late: He died of lung cancer in 1957.)

Later in 1950 two British investigators, Dr. Richard Doll and A. Bradford Hill, reported that their survey of lung-cancer patients at 20 London hospitals found fewer than 0.3 per cent of the victims to be nonsmokers. Then Dr. Doll and Hill followed the lives of some 40,000 British physicians for more than four years, comparing death rates and causes of deaths for smokers and nonsmokers. In 1956 the team concluded that, depending on the number of cigarettes smoked per day, smokers were seven to 24 times as likely to die of lung cancer as nonsmokers.

Scores of later studies, including the American Cancer

*Streaks of tars known to be a cause of cancer blacken the
lung tissue of a heavy cigarette smoker (below, right), in dramatic
contrast to the clean appearance of healthy lung cells (below,
left). The dark tissue is from a smoker who died of lung cancer.*

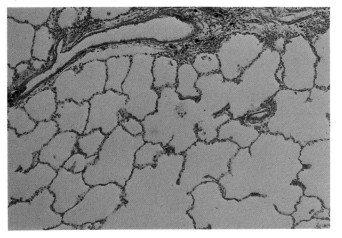 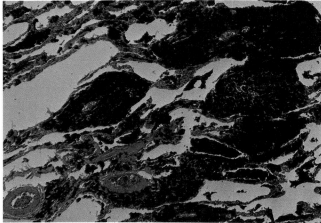

Society's mammoth Cancer Prevention Study, which was begun in 1959, confirmed and refined these findings. Astonishingly, in the confusing and often contentious world of statistical study and interpretation, not a single analysis has failed to show that lung-cancer victims consistently smoke more than people who do not get the disease. By contrast, population groups who do not smoke, such as Mormons and Seventh-day Adventists, have significantly lower rates of lung cancer.

By medical consensus, smokers who consume one to two packs of cigarettes a day are approximately 10 times as likely to develop lung cancer as nonsmokers. One out of every five heavy smokers—40 cigarettes a day or more—is fated to die of lung cancer. Lung cancer is the leading cause of cancer deaths among men, and in the mid-1980s it is expected to surpass breast cancer as the leading cause of cancer deaths among women. More than 100,000 Americans die from lung cancer each year; in Canada the toll is some 7,000; in Great Britain more than 30,000; in West Germany about 25,000.

Even more alarming, smoking has been shown to increase a person's risk not only of lung cancer but of emphysema, heart disease and a whole range of other afflictions. Pack-a-day cigarette smokers are nine times as likely as non-smokers to suffer mouth cancer, seven times as likely to get cancer of the larynx, six times as likely to contract cancer of

the esophagus and three times as likely to get bladder cancer.

Laboratory tests confirm the toxicity of cigarette smoke. Substances condensed from it—so-called tars—contain such chemicals as benzopyrene, nitrosamine and dibenzanthrocene. They are known carcinogens. Painted onto the skin of rabbits, mice and rats, they produce skin cancer; presumably they have a similar effect on human lung tissue. If the smoke is forced into dogs' breathing passages, the result is lung malignancies remarkably similar to human tumors.

Attempts to concoct ''safe'' cigarettes have met limited success. About half of the approximately 600 billion cigarettes sold annually in the United States contain 50 per cent less tar and nicotine than standard ones. These low-tar, low-nicotine brands are less harmful, but only to a limited degree. Dr. E. Cuyler Hammond of the American Cancer Society reported that men who smoked such cigarettes were from 17 to 21 per cent less likely to die of lung cancer than other cigarette smokers, and that women were from 38 to 43 per cent less likely.

Many cigarette smokers believe they can escape the risk of cancer, and particularly the risk of lung cancer, if they switch to smoking cigars or a pipe, because in theory they do not inhale. In fact, many converts to cigars or pipes do inhale some of the smoke and, puff for puff, cigar and pipe smoke contains as much tar and nicotine as cigarette smoke. And cigars and pipes bring the same risk as cigarettes of cancer of the esophagus, pharynx, mouth and lip.

Such evidence led health officials in many countries to launch antismoking campaigns. In Sweden no fewer than 16 different warnings are printed, on a rotating basis, on cigarette packages so that smokers do not become numbed to a single repeated appeal. A few countries, such as Finland, Norway and Singapore, have banned all cigarette advertising, and elsewhere partial bans control either the content of the advertisements or the media in which they may be used.

In the United States, the Surgeon General declared: ''Cigarette smoking is a health hazard of sufficient importance in the United States to warrant remedial action.'' Congress then ordered manufacturers to begin printing health warnings on every cigarette package, and cigarette advertise-ments were banned on American television and radio.

The antismoking efforts have proved effective. In 1964 about 52 per cent of American men and 32 per cent of women were smokers. Almost two decades later the figures had dropped to about 40 per cent for men and 30 per cent for women. Smoking trends in other Western countries show similar, if less dramatic, downturns.

Those who have forsworn cigarettes are the beneficiaries of a medical quirk: Although other cancer-causing substances remain in the body indefinitely and may bring on cancer decades after they were encountered, those implanted by smoking diminish rapidly in injurious effect. Ten to 15 years after giving up the habit, a reformed smoker faces a lung-cancer risk nearly as low as that of someone who has never smoked at all.

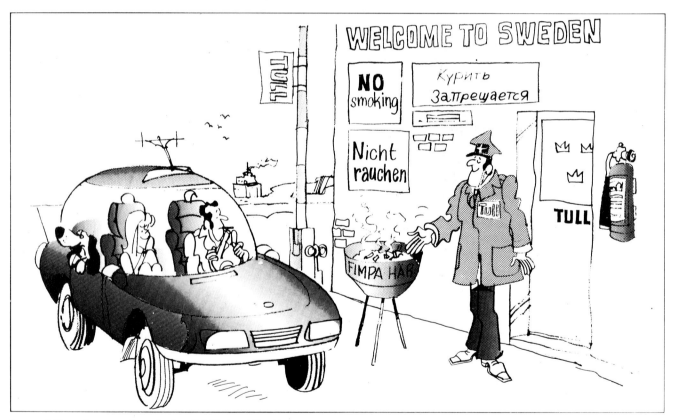

In a multilingual cartoon from the Swedish National Smoking and Health Association, visitors to a future Sweden are reminded that smoking is no longer allowed there. The association's program of education and lobbying, begun in 1973, has led to legal limits on tobacco advertising, warnings printed on packages, and proposed laws to restrict smoking in public places.

Still, millions of people the world over continue to smoke. Though per capita cigarette consumption has decreased, the total number of cigarettes smoked has gone up since the massive antismoking campaigns began. "We physicians and scientists are amazed," commented Dr. R. Lee Clark of the M. D. Anderson Hospital and Tumor Institute in Houston in 1980, "at the widespread disregard during the past 17 years of the proof of how to prevent lung cancer and other serious health problems by not inhaling tobacco smoke."

There are many reasons why so many people have either disregarded the scientists' proof or, if they accepted it, failed to take action on it. Politics and economics are involved. In many countries, entire regions depend on tobacco farming and cigarette manufacturing. But cigarettes themselves can gain a hold on smokers that is more insidious than any persuasion put forth by financial interests. Tobacco is addictive. It contains not only tars that are carcinogenic but also nicotine, a powerfully addictive drug. Cigarettes give many people an immense amount of psychological and physical pleasure. Some people smoke because that first rush of nicotine calms them. Others are stimulated. For still others, smoking is a means to curb appetite for food, to appear sophisticated or to gain the acceptance of peers.

How to stop smoking for good

The reasons for continuing to smoke pale beside those for stopping. And the number of people who persist in the habit should not obscure the achievement of the many who have given it up. Quitting may not be easy, but several different methods have been devised to help a smoker become a nonsmoker. The best way, one study demonstrated, is to stop cold, not gradually. Saul M. Shiffman and Dr. Murray E. Jarvik of the University of California at Los Angeles compared the two techniques on 40 volunteers who smoked. One group quit cold and remained abstinent for two weeks; the other group reduced normal cigarette consumption by an average of 60 per cent over the period. Four times a day, the subjects answered questionnaires about their withdrawal symptoms, including alertness and drowsiness, physical comfort and discomfort, and craving for tobacco.

Although the two groups initially reported comparably severe withdrawal symptoms, only the group that stopped abruptly experienced a rapid and notable lessening of such symptoms. "It may be," stated the researchers, "that the smoker who substantially reduces his cigarette smoking precipitates an abstinence syndrome no less severe than that in the completely abstinent smoker, yet perpetuates this syndrome by continuing to smoke."

Thus, cutting the habit gradually appears to make eventual quitting more difficult. "Craving," the scientists said, "leads to smoking, to craving, in a cycle of dependence."

To bolster the resolve to hold out against such cravings, one United States government agency suggests the following program:

● Set a target date for quitting. Birthdays, anniversaries, holidays, New Year's Day or the first day of vacation are favorites. Needless to say, stick to your target date.

● On the days before you quit, smoke more heavily than usual, overdosing on cigarettes and making the experience as distasteful as possible. Collect your cigarette butts from those days to serve as a reminder of smoking's filth.

● On the day you quit, throw away all cigarettes and matches. Hide lighters and ash trays. Visit the dentist and have your teeth cleaned to get rid of unsightly tobacco stains. Above all, stay busy—go to the movies, take a long walk, visit friends who do not smoke.

● For the first few days after quitting, spend as much time as possible in places where smoking is prohibited—libraries, museums, theaters. Avoid alcohol, coffee and other beverages you associate with smoking.

● If you miss the sensation of holding a cigarette, pick up a pencil, a paper clip or a string of beads and play with it. If you miss having something in your mouth, try toothpicks, sugarless gum or hard candy.

● If the urge to smoke strikes, brush your teeth or munch a low-calorie food such as a carrot, a pickle, a piece of celery or an apple.

● Plan celebrations to mark milestones on the road to smokelessness. After your first week, or month, or year without cigarettes, treat yourself to a movie, a sports event or

a pleasant dinner, using the money you will have saved.
● Above all, never allow yourself to think that "just one cigarette won't hurt." It will.

Many people who want to stop smoking benefit from outside help, and a number of programs have been set up. Some of them employ direct methods of altering behavior, aiming to make the smoker dislike the habit by associating it with something very unpleasant, such as electric shocks *(pages 51-53)*. Hypnosis, in which a therapist instills in the subconscious the idea that smoking is harmful, is used by others. The most popular programs use group counseling, bringing together small numbers of smokers for regular meetings to discuss means of quitting and compare experiences. The effectiveness of any of these techniques remains to be proved —some claim success rates of 10 to 20 per cent, others 70 per cent. All of the techniques work for some people—and whatever works is a valuable step in avoiding cancer.

Closely related to tobacco as an inducer of cancer—and equally avoidable—is alcohol. Alone it does not seem to bring malignancies, and in moderation it can be beneficial to health, relieving stress. But when consumed in large quantities, it greatly increases the lethal effect of tobacco, acting as a so-called co-carcinogen. A man who smokes and is also a heavy drinker—consuming three martinis or six glasses of beer a day—increases his chances of getting cancer; he has a risk of oral cancer 15 times higher than a teetotaling non-smoking man. Similar synergisms exist for cancers of the esophagus and larynx, and possibly of the bladder and liver. (Alcohol never comes in direct contact with the lungs, so it does not increase the risk of lung cancer.)

The most plausible explanation for the carcinogenic effect of alcohol and tobacco is that the two reinforce each other's irritation of tissues in body passageways. A rival explanation hinges on the observation that heavy drinkers suffer deficiencies of key nutrients because alcohol reduces appetite.

Food: cause and preventive

Eating patterns may strongly affect the risk of developing cancer. What you eat certainly is within your control. Thus, by eliminating smoking, cutting down on alcohol—and eating a healthful, nutritious diet—you can reduce your risk of many cancers. A proper diet may help reduce the cancer risk by 30 per cent.

Some things you consume almost certainly bring on cancer. Others may prevent it. A number of vitamins and minerals, for example, have been touted as cancer preventives, and there is evidence that a few might be effective. But most of this evidence is indirect. It is based on studies that show that certain cancers are more prevalent among populations lacking in specific dietary elements—thereby suggesting the value of a food component by demonstrating harm attributed to a lack of it. One study linked a pocket of mouth and esophageal cancer among Scandinavian women to an iron deficiency. Another indicated that people in such landlocked countries as Austria and Switzerland—where iodine-rich seafoods are scarce—exhibit unusually high rates of cancer of the thyroid gland, an organ known to require iodine.

Similar studies implicate a lack of vitamin A. The London-based International Cancer Research Fund reported a five-year investigation of 16,000 British men, 86 of whom developed cancer. Blood samples from the 86 were compared with those from men of similar age and habits who had not developed cancer. The men with the lowest vitamin A levels were more than twice as likely to develop cancer—especially cancer of the lung—as men with higher quantities of the substance in their blood.

Vitamin C, heralded as an antidote for the common cold, has also been claimed to ward off cancer. Studies of stomach-cancer patients in particular show that they include a disproportionate number who consumed diets low in vitamin C. But the most tantalizing report in favor of a connection between vitamin C and cancer came from a Scottish doctor working with the American Nobel laureate chemist Linus Pauling, a champion of the medicinal value of vitamin C.

In 1974 Pauling and Dr. Ewan Cameron of the Vale of Leven District General Hospital reported on a study of a group of 1,100 cancer patients known to be near death. The treatments they had been getting were discontinued as pointless, but 100 of them were given large doses of vitamin C—more than 150 times the amount healthy people require. Al-

Learning to hate a hazardous habit

"I have stopped smoking now and then," said author Mark Twain, "to pulverize those critics who said I was a slave to my habits and couldn't break my bonds." Twain never did quit for good, smoking and coughing to the end, but like millions of others who tried to kick the habit and failed, he might have succeeded with help from a stop-smoking program. Many kinds of aid are offered—some free, some costing hundreds of dollars—by a variety of sponsors, including cancer-fighting societies, church and community groups, and commercial clinics. Their success rates are hard to evaluate, but some claim that as many as 70 per cent of their graduates stop smoking for at least a year.

Nearly all programs work to change a person's psychological as well as physical addiction to tobacco, though their means differ greatly. Some programs use hypnosis in an attempt to supplement will power; others consist mainly of lecture classes. The Seventh-day Adventist Church brings smokers together for a five-day retreat where they must stop smoking immediately—tobacco is banned.

Techniques of behavioral psychology are used by clinics of the Schick Center for the Control of Smoking. The center's "aversion conditioning" links smoking to an unpleasant stimulus—an electric shock or a bad taste or smell—thus associating the once-enjoyable experience with something negative. In individual sessions, each patient puffs without inhaling while receiving mild shocks, then chain-smokes briefly and inhales rapidly to the point of discomfort without receiving the zaps *(right and the following pages)*. For six weeks he also attends meetings on nutrition, relaxation and behavior modification—all to help him remain a nonsmoker for life.

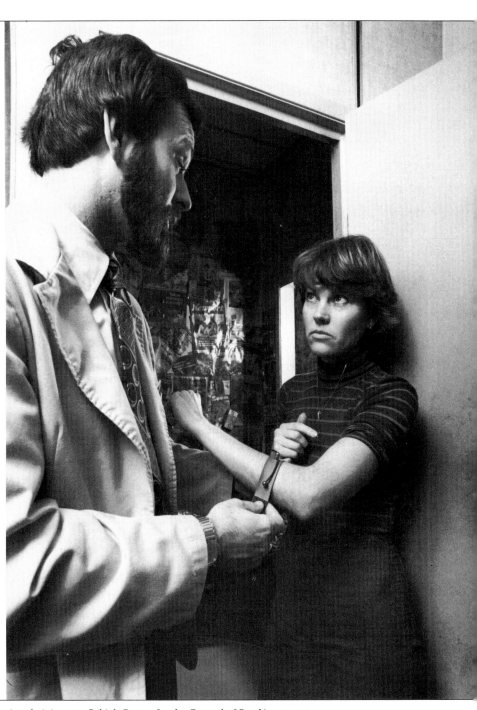

A technician at a Schick Center for the Control of Smoking straps an electrode called a faradic stimulator—from "faraday," a measurement of electricity—to the arm of a woman about to begin five hour-long aversion therapy sessions. For the five days preceding this session, she recorded the number of cigarettes she smoked and eliminated as many as possible.

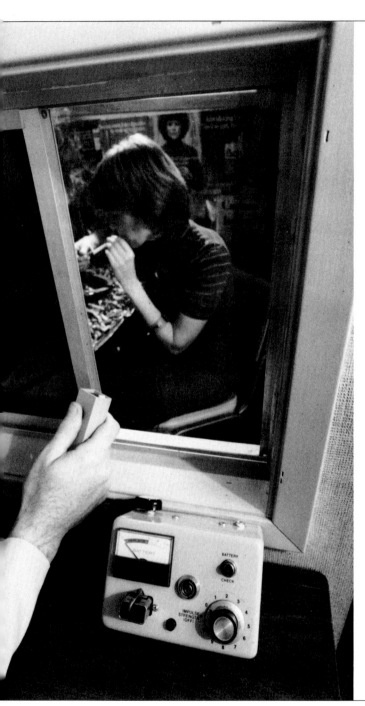

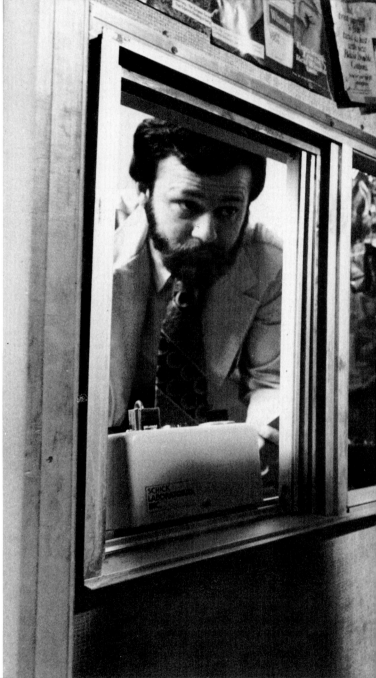

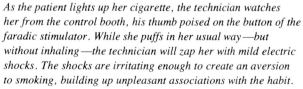

As the patient lights up her cigarette, the technician watches her from the control booth, his thumb poised on the button of the faradic stimulator. While she puffs in her usual way—but without inhaling—the technician will zap her with mild electric shocks. The shocks are irritating enough to create an aversion to smoking, building up unpleasant associations with the habit.

In another stage of her session, the patient smokes three cigarettes, inhaling every six seconds until she becomes uncomfortable and wants to stop smoking. The technician does not deliver shocks during this period. Further reinforcing her growing distaste for smoking are advertisements on the walls, and ash trays overflowing with half-smoked cigarettes.

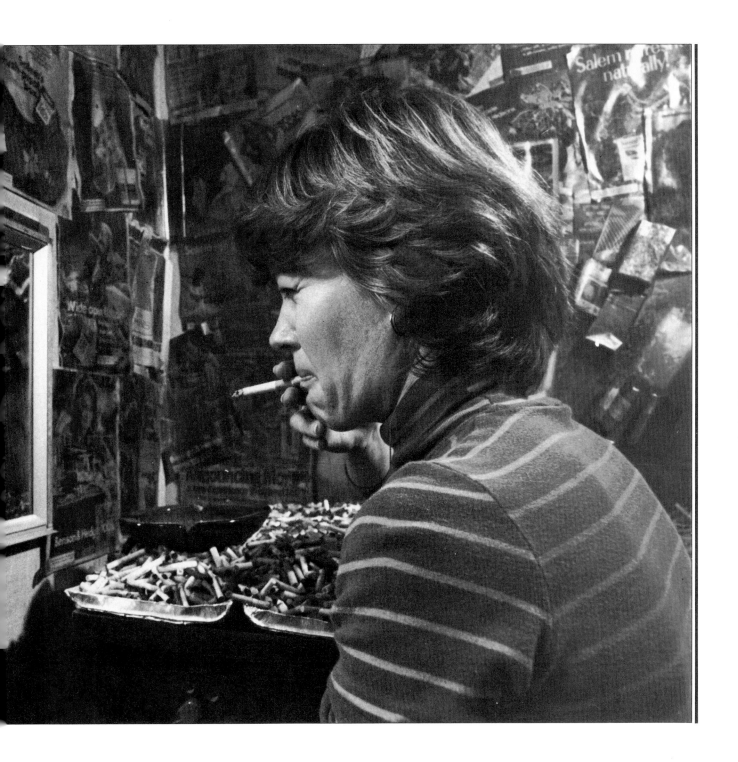

though none of the patients survived, the lives of those receiving vitamin C were extended; following cessations of other treatment, they lived an average of 4.2 times as long as the controls. However, five years later a similar investigation at the Mayo Clinic in Rochester, Minnesota, failed to duplicate the results of Pauling and Dr. Cameron.

The evidence needed to prove an unquestionable link between vitamin and mineral deficiencies and cancer is not yet in. And attempting to prevent cancer with huge doses of mineral supplements or vitamin pills can be dangerous: Excess vitamin A can cause blurred vision or blindness, and liver and bone damage; vitamin C in large doses can promote the formation of kidney stones, among other effects.

More innocuous is another food component often recommended as a cancer antidote: fiber, the indigestible bulk or roughage in many fruits, vegetables and whole-grain cereal products such as bran. Its role was noted in East Africa by Denis Burkitt—the Irish surgeon who discovered the virus-caused jaw cancer bearing his name *(pages 104-105)*. Burkitt, whose espousal of fiber earned him the nickname the Bran Man, became, he said, "acutely conscious that a high proportion of the beds in any Western hospital are filled with patients suffering from diseases which are rare or unknown in the rest of the world." Cancer of the colon, Burkitt noted, was second only to lung cancer as a killer in Western Europe and North America, but was virtually nonexistent in East Africa. The disparity, he concluded, arose from the Africans' higher intake of fiber—as much as three ounces per day. Westerners, who process most of the fiber out of their foods, consume on the average about one ounce per day. Fiber absorbs liquids, and because it is indigestible, it passes through the digestive system quickly, presumably flushing carcinogens out of the body before they can do much harm.

The Bran Man's theory is not universally accepted. Animals fed high-fiber diets develop colon cancer at virtually the same rate as those on low-fiber diets. The Japanese, who have a very low incidence of colon cancer, do not consume a diet notably high in fiber. And high-fiber intake is not the only dietary difference between East Africans and Westerners. Westerners' heavy consumption of animal fats might explain the disparity in the two groups' colon-cancer rates.

Considerable research has focused on the abundance of animal fat in the Western diet, not the absence of fiber, as the key factor in extraordinary regional differences in colon cancer. In many Western countries, fats—from milk and cheese, fried foods, and particularly from beef, pork and lamb—contribute up to 40 per cent of a person's average daily intake of calories. In the East African countries studied by Burkitt—and in many other countries with low colon-cancer rates, such as Japan, Thailand and India—fats contribute a mere 12 per cent of the average caloric intake. But when people from those countries migrate to the West and take up the high-fat diet, their colon-cancer rates gradually approach those of Westerners.

Much research links high-fat diets with cancer. Among people with colon cancer, such diets are associated with an increase in the bile acids formed in the liver to help process fats. And when such acids are injected into the colons of rats, they hasten the formation of tumors caused by other carcinogens. Cancers of the breast, prostate gland, ovaries, lining of the uterus, and pancreas also may be related to high-fat diets, apparently because such diets alter the balance of hormones that, among other things, regulate growth and development. Stimulated by a surge of a hormone, a tumor begins to grow.

Most authorities believe that another cause of cancer is foods that have been heavily salted and smoked. The Japanese, whose diet is low in fats, consume large quantities of salty pickles and soybean sauces, and of smoked fish. Although their low-fat diet appears to protect them from colon cancer, their salty, smoked foods evidently contribute to a stomach-cancer rate eight times higher than that in the United States, where such delicacies are less popular.

These findings, some tentative and some fairly certain, have been translated into prudent advice by experts at the government-supported American Health Foundation:

● Consume a generous amount of fiber, available in fresh fruits and vegetables and unrefined grains—a bowl of all-bran cereal or eight slices of whole-grain bread each day.

● Cut down on fatty foods: cheese, whole milk, beef, pork, lamb and any fried foods.

● Keep alcohol consumption moderate—one or two drinks per day at the most.

● Avoid salty foods—including heavily marinated preparations, pickles and salty snacks such as peanuts and pretzels—and use less salt at the table.

Perilous additives

The cancer danger—or protection—presented by food generally comes from the foodstuff itself or from traditional methods of preparing it, such as smoking or salting. But a new source of concern arose with the introduction into commercially processed foods of additives, many of them previously unknown chemicals synthesized in the laboratory rather than natural materials that people have been consuming over the millennia. They serve a variety of purposes. Some make the food more appetizing by improving flavor, color or texture; others are disease preventives that provide essential health protection.

A few additives have been identified as clearly dangerous carcinogens, and banned from foods. But a number of others are under suspicion though not convicted. In many cases the danger is slight and the value of the additive great. Thus protection against possibly carcinogenic additives requires fine judgment, a delicate balancing of risk against benefit. Additive-free meals can be prepared, either by processing at home or by searching out commercial products that contain none. But forgoing additives may make it necessary to forgo some flavor, accept an unappetizing color—or risk dangerous contamination. For example, hot dogs without sodium nitrite, a coloring and preservative that can help induce cancer, are gray instead of the familiar red and they must be freshly and carefully prepared—the lack of nitrite may permit growth of the bacteria that cause deadly botulism.

A subtler judgment is called for in the case of another type of food additive, artificial sweeteners. Two synthetics, cyclamate and saccharin, are of inestimable value to people—diabetics and the overweight—who ought not satisfy the human craving for sweets with sugar's concentrated-carbohydrate calories. Both synthetic compounds have been implicated in cancer. Cyclamate, introduced in the 1950s, was found to cause tumors in rats. In a study sponsored in the late 1960s by cyclamate producers, 240 laboratory rats were fed a cyclamate-rich diet for 16 months. Much to the industry's chagrin, four of the rats came down with bladder tumors and four others with suspicious lesions.

Experts were called in to examine the results. The prestigious British medical journal *Lancet,* in a wry paraphrase of wartime Prime Minister Winston Churchill, stated: ''Never have so many pathologists been summoned to opine on so few lesions from so humble a species as the laboratory rat.'' But because cyclamate was a possible carcinogen, it was banned in the United States in 1969. Later tests of cyclamate proved negative, and its exclusion may have been a mistake.

Then in 1977 the other artificial sweetener, saccharin—a compound in wide use for a century—came under attack. Researchers at the Canadian government's Health Protection Branch in Ottawa released the results of an extensive animal study. Of 100 rats fed huge amounts of saccharin (5 per cent of their total diet), three developed bladder tumors. In another test group of 100 rats, exposed to similarly high doses both in their mothers' wombs and throughout their lives, 14 developed bladder tumors.

A few weeks later a second Canadian experiment reported even more disturbing results on humans. It compared 632 bladder-cancer patients with a similar number without the disease and found that high intake of artificial sweeteners, principally saccharin, was associated with a 60 per cent greater bladder-cancer risk among men.

The Canadian government banned the sweetener and the U.S. Food and Drug Administration announced its intention to do the same. Shoppers raced to supermarkets to snap up popular products containing the substance. The public outcry in the United States was loud. In response to the public objections—and to scientific criticism of the Canadian tests—the United States Congress ordered the intended ban postponed. Thus arose one of the more curious paradoxes in the fight against cancer. Cyclamate was legally prohibited as carcinogenic in the United States but saccharin was not. In the next-door-neighbor country of Canada, saccharin was prohibited in food and beverages but cyclamate was not.

With hands inserted into gloves of a sealed enclosure, a technician measures out a substance to be tested for cancer-causing danger. In this Ames assay—named after its inventor, Dr. Bruce Ames of Berkeley—the substance is mixed with Salmonella bacteria. If it causes genetic changes in the bacteria, there is a 90 per cent chance it will cause cancer in human beings.

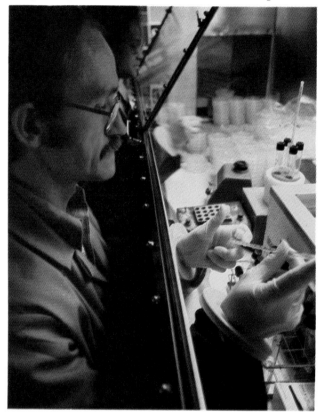

The prudent course is clear but may not be easy to follow: Consume as little artificial sweetener as possible. The danger from using small amounts seems slight. However, many people trying to control their weight—particularly children—consume large amounts of it in prepared foods; the child who drinks several bottles of diet soda a day is not unusual. And each 12-ounce bottle of diet soda contains $1/200$ ounce of saccharin—a very small amount that adds up to a large one if the soda habit continues over the years.

Weighing risks in medicines

An individual can choose the foods he wants to eat and avoid others. He has less power over other possible carcinogens he ingests in medicines prescribed by a physician. Some drugs have been found—belatedly—to be potent causes of cancer.

Among those arousing the most concern are hormones—synthetic versions of the natural substances governing a variety of body functions. They have been used to treat such ills as menopausal complaints, and they are the principal ingredients in birth-control pills.

From the mid-1940s until the mid-1960s, the synthetic female hormone diethylstilbestrol, or DES, was prescribed to prevent miscarriage for an estimated two million pregnant American women. Its effectiveness for this purpose is now in doubt, but by 1970 another effect became alarmingly apparent. In 1966 Drs. Howard Ulfelder and Arthur S. Herbst of Boston's Massachusetts General Hospital examined a 16-year-old girl whose complaint—vaginal bleeding—they diagnosed as a rare cancer of the vagina. Over the next four years seven other young women, all with the same ailment, came in to see the physicians. Drs. Herbst and Ulfelder were at first at a loss to account for the peculiar outbreak. By exhaustive inquiry into medical records, however, they and their colleagues discovered that each of the girls had been born to mothers who had been given DES while pregnant.

Investigations elsewhere found that some sons born to DES mothers were deficient in sperm, a sign of sterility. DES was banned as a medicine for pregnant women and also as a supplement to cattle feed, in which it had been mixed to induce rapid weight gain. However, the harm done in the past cannot be undone; women who know or suspect their mothers were given DES should get frequent examinations for signs of vaginal cancer, which is curable if treated promptly.

Other hormones are still used. Female hormones slightly different in composition from DES are frequently prescribed to alleviate the palpitations, hot flashes and depression that often accompany menopause. These drugs, too, involve risks. One study at the University of Southern California found that a woman who begins taking such hormone supplements at age 50 doubles her risk of developing breast cancer by age 75. And numerous studies have shown a fivefold-to-tenfold increase in the risk of cancer of the uterine lining among postmenopausal women who took hormones.

The use of hormones for menopausal ailments is minuscule compared with their consumption in contraceptive pills—80 million women in the world take them almost daily during many of their childbearing years. Some cancer researchers fear that the Pill may in due course bring an increased risk of breast cancer. Paradoxically, other specialists believe it may provide some protection against that very same ailment—they suspect that the hormone promotes the growth of some types of tumors but inhibits others.

Because the potential risk from contraceptives is so widespread, considerable research has been devoted to gauge the hazard. One extensive investigation, a 10-year study of 16,000 women by the Kaiser Permanente Medical Center in California, was generally reassuring. Though use of the Pill seemed to increase slightly the risk of lung cancer among smokers and of a type of skin cancer among sunburn victims, the effect was minute. "The risks of oral contraceptive use," concluded the scientists, "appear to be negligible." But they cautioned that women choosing this method of birth control "must weigh the pros and cons among uncertainties."

Why to avoid a fashionable tan

In contrast to such cancer hazards as drugs, foods and tobacco, which are at least partially subject to individual control, are two others that many people accept almost fatalistically as dangers that can be regulated only by national—or international—law. They are the various forms of energetic rays called radiation and the pollution of the environment by chemicals. Yet even these carcinogens can often be avoided.

Perhaps the most feared cause of cancer is the many types of radiation. The effects of nuclear warfare, seen only in Hiroshima and Nagasaki, are disastrous. Peacetime dangers arise in radiation from the sun, from medical X-rays, from the soil and from nuclear power plants.

Sunlight produces skin cancer because its ultraviolet rays penetrate the skin. They damage the skin's elastic fibers, altering the structure of epidermal cells and making them cancerous. Not everyone is equally susceptible. Risk depends on the amount of natural pigment, or melanin, present. Dark-skinned people have plenty of melanin and are relatively protected from the sun's rays; fair-haired, blue-eyed, light-skinned people have less and are more vulnerable.

The most common forms of the disease—so-called superficial skin cancers—manifest themselves as brown patches or scaly areas. Some 95 per cent of all cases are curable, usually through routine treatments in a doctor's office, but the skin may be left discolored or scarred. Said one famous skin-cancer victim, Ernest Hemingway, to a youngster who asked why he wore a beard: "Kid, if you had skin cancer, you'd grow a beard too." One skin cancer, malignant melanoma, is deadly; the risk is greatest in the direct sunlight of semitropical areas, especially if normally light-skinned people try to get deep tans. In such sunny areas as the American state of Arizona and Queensland, Australia *(pages 13-15)*, the melanoma death rate is about 14 per 100,000 population.

Health authorities decry the vogue for tanned skin. They urge caution outdoors, not only in the tropics and semitropics but also anywhere in the mountains, where thin air transmits more ultraviolet rays, and near water, which multiplies radiation's effects. They urge that, when you are outdoors, you:
● Wear light clothing and a hat, reducing the area of the body you expose to the sun.
● Use lotions that block ultraviolet rays. The best sunscreens contain para-aminobenzoic acid, or PABA, and are graded for their sun-blocking properties. The grade numbers—2 to 15—are printed on the containers; the higher the number, the greater the protection.
● Apply lotion often, especially after going in the water.
● Do not use baby oil, mineral oil or olive oil. These can actually magnify the sun's rays.
● Be especially cautious during midday hours, when the sun's rays are most damaging.
● Beware of cloudy days. Ultraviolet rays penetrate clouds.

Less easily managed are other kinds of radiation—the radioactive types that come from X-rays and many natural and man-made atomic sources. More than half of a person's annual exposure to radioactivity is simply an unavoidable consequence of living—the result of background emissions from rocks, soil and the sun (which sends out atomic rays in addition to ultraviolet light).

Since its discovery, radiation has been known to cause cancer. Many early experimenters developed skin cancer.

A crusader called "Dr. Asbestos"

Soon after chest specialist Irving Selikoff opened a medical clinic in Paterson, New Jersey, in 1953, he detected a curious pattern of disease. Fifteen of his first paients had serious lung ailments, some later developing into cancers, and all 15 were employed by the city's Union Asbestos and Rubber Company. Intrigued, Dr. Selikoff set out to uncover the connection. What followed was a single-minded crusade that led Dr. Selikoff to start the Environmental Sciences Laboratory at New York City's Mount Sinai Medical Center, earned him the nickname "Dr. Asbestos," and provided much of the evidence implicating asbestos as a cause of cancer.

Part of that evidence came from a 1974 study of Thetford Mines, Quebec *(right),* an asbestos mining and milling town of 20,000. There, in a survey of 1,200 living and deceased asbestos workers, Dr. Selikoff and a Mount Sinai team uncovered a lung-cancer death rate more than double the Canadian national average.

Thanks to such research at Thetford Mines and elsewhere, many governments—including those of Canada and the United States—placed controls on asbestos manufacturing and banned the insulating material in new construction. "Unfortunately," said Dr. Selikoff, "we're going to be paying the price of our past mistakes for many years."

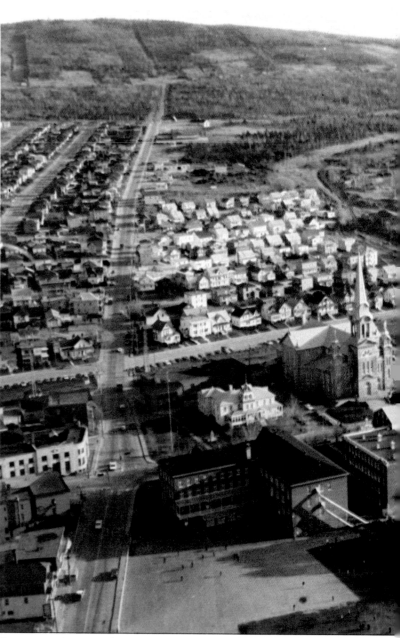

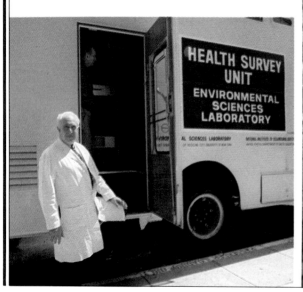

Dr. Irving J. Selikoff prepares to step aboard a mobile laboratory used by one of his research teams. In addition to the study at Thetford Mines, Dr. Selikoff and his teams have conducted investigations of job-related disease all over North America.

Steam spews from an asbestos mining and milling operation in the town of Thetford Mines, Quebec, site of the oldest asbestos mine in North America. Visible behind the plant building are pyramids of poisonous asbestos residue and an open-pit asbestos mine. Both the residues and the open-pit operation are health hazards located scarcely a mile away from the center of the town.

A clamp on his nose and a hose pressed to his mouth, an asbestos worker exhales into a machine that measures how much air his lungs can hold and how fast he can exhale. Low lung capacity is an indication of asbestos damage.

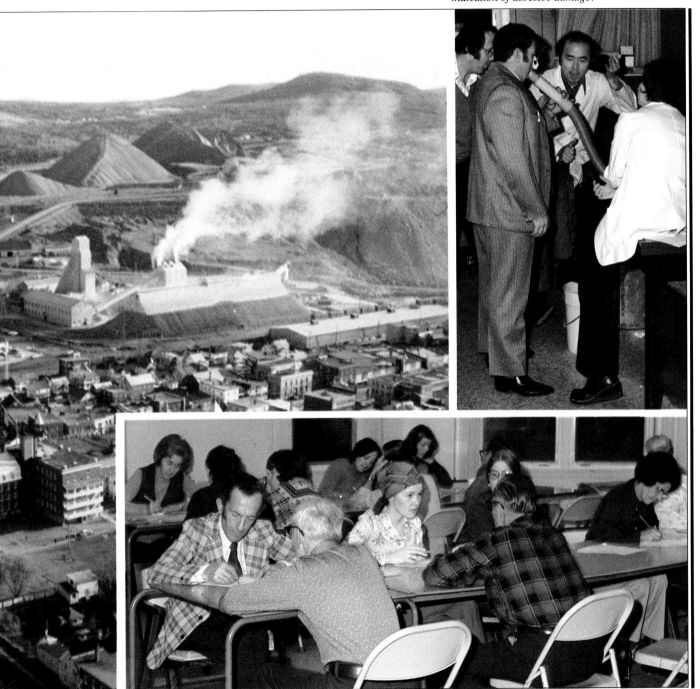

Thetford Mines workers seated at long tables complete detailed job- and health-history questionnaires. The information, together with test results and mortality figures, helps researchers measure health risks for various asbestos-industry jobs.

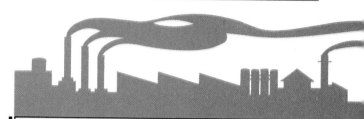

Marie Curie, who with her husband, Pierre, discovered radium, died of cancer; so did their daughter, Irène, and son-in-law, Frederic Joliot, both scientists who worked with the elder Curies. Cancer has long been recognized as an occupational hazard of radiologists. Yet these tragically acquired lessons are repeatedly forgotten. In the 1910s and 1920s, women who painted radium onto luminous watch dials in a New Jersey factory pointed their brushes with their lips; no fewer than 71 died of cancer, primarily of the bone and jaw.

As late as the 1950s doctors in the Chicago area treated children for respiratory ailments by bombarding their thymus glands and tonsils with X-rays—a disastrous mistake that made the subjects, years later, susceptible to cancer of the thyroid, the gland that is exceptionally vulnerable to radiation's cancer-causing effects. During the same period, shoe stores all across the United States used X-ray devices to fit shoes; no one knows how much harm was done.

How much radiation may be tolerable depends on several factors. Radiation has a cumulative effect over the years: The impact of today's exposure is added to earlier exposures. The body has some ability to neutralize the effect of minor X-rays, and a number of small exposures spread over the years are not as harmful as a single large dose.

Exposure to radiation is measured in units called rads, the amount of radiation absorbed by body tissues. A chest X-ray delivers .02 to .06 rad, the average dental X-ray up to 10 times as much but to a much smaller area. Scientists estimate that the average person receives .2 rad each year, with no apparent harm. Some people receive more: Because residents of mile-high Denver live slightly closer to the sun, they take in about .06 rad per year more radiation than do inhabitants of London. Similarly, airline crews are exposed a trifle more as they jet along at 38,000 feet. But neither residents of Denver nor air crews exhibit unusually high cancer rates.

The atomic rays from natural sources—the sun, soil and rocks—are so few that they are not believed bothersome. Concern centers on the similar rays that are man-made, particularly in X-ray machines and nuclear power plants.

Although the benefits of X-rays are immeasurable—medicine has no comparable means of seeing into the body's

A multitude of carcinogens on the job

Almost everyone is exposed to something at work that might cause cancer. Even a coffee break could be hazardous, for coffee drinking has been implicated in cancer of the bladder. In any sampling of occupations linked to cancer, some on-the-job dangers are so obvious they are often overlooked, such as the skin cancer risked by sailors and farmers, who must spend their days outdoors exposed to the sun's ultraviolet rays. The danger in other jobs is less obvious. Vintners, for instance, were found to be susceptible to cancers of the liver, lung or skin. The cause, it turned out, is an arsenic insecticide used in some wine-growing areas, such as Germany's Moselle River regions, to spray the grapes.

Some industries—such as mining and textiles—have long been linked to a variety of cancers. Iron miners risk larynx and lung cancers from exposure to iron oxide, one of the principal ores. Gold miners in Zimbabwe and hard-rock miners in America are, like vintners, exposed to arsenic compounds, which are an unwanted component of the ores. In the textile industry, bladder cancer strikes many dyers who use substances known as aromatic amines (beta-naphthylamine, auramine, magenta and others). Underwater construction workers may contract bone cancer from long periods of activity with a limited oxygen supply, while textile printers working with dyes containing cadmium are prone to kidney, lung or prostate cancers.

The variety of jobs that exist within some industries often makes it difficult to pinpoint cancer causes. Studies can be further complicated when booming industries such as the insulation business bring on new hazards. Even in an old trade a small change can create a cancer puzzle. Why, after centuries, did cases of bladder cancer crop up among Japanese kimono painters? It was finally discovered that cancer-inducing benzidine had been substituted for the traditional vegetable materials in the paint used by the artists. And like American radium-dial painters of the 1920s, who figured in the classic case of cancer detective work, the kimono painters habitually pointed their brushes with their lips, thereby ingesting a lethal substance.

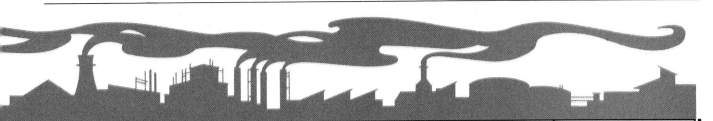

OCCUPATION	Suspected cause of cancer	Types of cancer	Incubation period (years)
AUTOMOBILE MECHANIC	Petroleum products	Larynx, lung, nasal passages, scrotum, skin	12-30
CARPENTER	Wood dusts	Nasal passages and sinuses	30-40
CHIMNEY SWEEP	Soot and other coal products	Bladder, larynx, lung, scrotum, skin	9-23
DYER	Aromatic amines Benzene	Bladder Leukemia	13-30 6-14
FARMER, SAILOR	Ultraviolet rays	Skin	Varies by skin color and skin texture
LEATHER WORKER	Leather dusts	Bladder, nasal passages, sinuses	40-50
MINER	Arsenic Asbestos Coal Iron oxide Uranium	Liver, lung, skin Lung Bladder, larynx, lung, scrotum, skin Larynx, lung Bone, lung, skin	10 or more 4-50 9-23 Not known 10-15
PAINTER	Benzene	Leukemia	6-14
POTTER	Chromium	Larynx, lung, nasal passages, sinuses	15-25
RUBBER WORKER	Aromatic amines Vinyl chloride	Bladder Brain, liver	13-30 20-30
SHOEMAKER	Benzene	Leukemia	6-14
TEXTILE PRINTER	Cadmium	Kidney, lung, prostate	Not known
UNDERWATER CONSTRUCTION WORKER	Lack of oxygen	Bone	Not known
VINTNER	Arsenic	Liver, lung, skin	10 or more
WELDER	Cadmium	Kidney, lung, prostate	Not known

innards and, ironically, sometimes no better way of killing cancer cells—control over exposure is universally urged. The limits have been progressively tightened over the years. Until 1980, for example, the American Cancer Society recommended a routine annual chest X-ray to detect lung cancer for adults who smoke heavily. Then the society became convinced the benefits gained were outweighed by the slight additional risk induced by the X-rays, and it deleted the chest X-ray from its suggested routine examination.

Although X-rays are administered only on the orders of a physician or dentist, the patient must accept some responsibility for controlling his exposure to them. The following precautions are generally recommended:
- Be sure that any X-ray is absolutely necessary. Often a previous X-ray will serve. Surveys have revealed that almost a third of all X-rays contribute no new information.
- Be sure the dentist or doctor covers areas outside the X-ray field—especially genitals—with a protective apron.
- Be especially careful whenever a child is involved. Children are at least five times more sensitive to radiation-induced cancer than adults.
- Pregnant women should not submit to X-rays except in an emergency. Exposure of the fetus to X-rays increases the vulnerability of the child to cancer.

More frightening and controversial than diagnostic X-rays is radiation from nuclear power plants. They release small amounts of radiation into the atmosphere and into river water used for cooling, but many experts believe the carcinogenic effect of this contamination is less than that of the smoke from coal-burning power plants. The real danger is posed by the possibility of a catastrophic accident that would release large amounts of radiation. Such an accident is considered very unlikely—how unlikely depends on the expert making the calculations and his attitude toward nuclear power.

One major accident, the March 1979 spill at the Three Mile Island plant in Pennsylvania, was serious but not catastrophic. For nearly two weeks, the world watched tensely while scientists struggled to gain control over a crippled reactor. After several valves failed, radioactive gas was released into the atmosphere. The maximum radiation received by anyone in the immediate area was about .1 rad—but that is one half the average person's annual dose. One expert suggested that the mishap might account over a 30-year period for one additional case of cancer in the vicinity and one additional death from it. At least a generation must pass before his estimate can be evaluated.

The occupational hazards

The only defense against danger from nuclear power plants is political action—or moving away if one is built near your home. Similarly limited options also apply to most environmental pollution, whether it affects only workers on a job or spreads over large parts of a country.

Ever since Percivall Pott reported in the 18th Century on the unduly high incidence of scrotal cancer among chimney sweeps *(Chapter 1),* people have been aware that workers in certain jobs run greater-than-normal cancer risks. As scientists have discovered new materials and compounds, manufacturers have rushed them to the marketplace. It may take 20 to 30 years to find out if they are harmful, and many substances become immensely valuable to society before danger is established. For instance, asbestos, which causes lung cancer, has saved untold lives through its use as a fire retardant and as a component of auto brake linings. Vinyl chloride gas not only provides a host of everyday items—phonograph records, furniture, food packages and babies' pacifiers—but it is indispensable in making lifesaving medical tubing and blood bags. Finished products based on vinyl chloride pose no known health hazards, but vinyl chloride workers face a 200-fold increased risk of liver cancer.

Often, however, dangerous chemicals spread far beyond the site of original use. Tons of wastes daily are spewed into the air, dumped into waters and buried underground. Farmers use pesticides to protect their crops and animals, but the chemicals, by definition deadly, infiltrate air, water supplies and forage, eventually to be consumed by humans.

Comparisons of relatively pollution-free rural areas to cities plagued by significant air pollution indicate the danger of environmental contamination. In a British study, conducted in 1957 by Dr. Percy Stocks, residents of "highly polluted'' Liverpool were found to suffer significantly higher rates of lung cancer than people who lived in "cleaner" North Wales. A recent study of United States communities where copper, lead or zinc smelters are located also suggested a connection between lung cancer and air pollution: Death rates from lung cancer were 15 to 17 per cent higher than normal in those areas. The difference presumably was due to arsenic released into the air by the smelters.

The case against specific water pollutants is generally less well documented, though one study suggested a surprising—and ironic—cancer connection. The President's Council on Environmental Quality reported in 1981 that Americans who drink water chlorinated to kill disease germs—a process hailed as one of the "major health advances of this century"—may bear a 13 to 93 per cent greater risk of rectal, colon and bladder cancer than those who drink well water.

The sea of carcinogens in which everyone must live is frightening. It has caused many people to make absurd efforts to avoid every substance or situation that has ever been accused of promoting cancer. Such extreme cancerphobia is counterproductive, "as serious to society," said *The New England Journal of Medicine,* "as it is to the individual—and morally more devastating."

When you are confronted with the possibility of cancers whose true cause is as yet unknown or to which your exposure is difficult to control, there are admittedly few preventive measures you can take. But avoiding carcinogens is not the only—or necessarily the best—safeguard. Learning how to spot cancer's early signs may be much more important. Early detection is paramount if cancer is to be cured.

To help people spot cancer early, the American Cancer Society has formulated what it calls the "seven warning signals" *(right, top).* Finding any one of them should call for an immediate examination by a doctor.

A change in bowel or bladder habits, for instance, or any unusual bleeding or discharge from the genital, urinary or digestive tract could signal a malignancy of the reproductive, urinary or gastrointestinal system. Severe indigestion or difficulty in swallowing could indicate, among other things,

Any of the seven signs listed in this photodiagram may warn of the onset of cancer. In themselves, the signs are ambiguous— a cough and hoarseness, for example, might be caused by a cold. But if any of them arises abruptly and persists, consult a doctor; detecting the site of a cancer before the disease invades other areas increases the patient's chance for a cure.

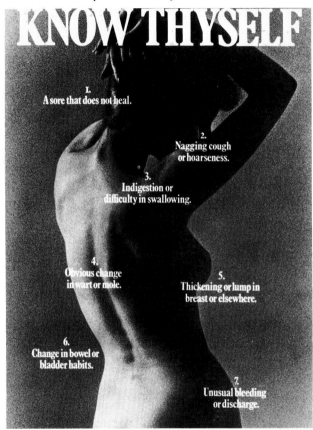

Know yourself. Know your body. Know the seven ways it warns you of changes that might mean cancer. If you have a warning signal, see your doctor promptly.
American Cancer Society

cancer of the throat, esophagus or stomach. A nagging cough might signal lung cancer, while a thickening or lump in the breast or elsewhere might mean a tumor in the affected area. A persistent sore or a change in a wart or mole could be a hint of a developing skin cancer.

For women, monthly breast self-examination—doctors refer to it as BSE—is essential *(pages 64-69).* It takes only a few minutes and it is the best means available for catching potential tumors early. Most women never detect any changes, and eight out of 10 lumps that are noticed prove harmless. But performing BSE faithfully saves lives. ✳

Breast self-examination: simple and sure

One out of every 11 women will suffer from breast cancer. The threat is subtle and insidious—a cancerous tumor may lie dormant and painless for years before being discovered—but it can and must be detected quickly. In the early stages, so long as the tumor grows no bigger than a marble and has not spread to other parts of the body, breast cancer is readily cured—80 to 90 per cent of the cases are successfully treated. But the longer the malignancy remains unnoticed and untreated, the greater the likelihood that it will spread and the less the likelihood that it can be eradicated.

The life-or-death responsibility for detecting breast cancer early falls primarily on each woman herself. Fortunately, it is a task she can easily manage. By regularly examining her own breasts—a simple procedure that requires only a large mirror and 10 minutes of time—she can detect warning signals soon enough for cure.

The main points to check, keyed by color in the picture opposite, are listed at right. Women who menstruate should conduct an examination each month, during the week after menstrual flow stops; nonmenstruating women—including not only those past menopause but also younger women who are pregnant or nursing—should examine their breasts the first day of each month.

The examination, illustrated in step-by-step photographs on the following pages, has two phases: visual and tactile. For both, a woman must know the normal characteristics of her own breasts, so that she can detect even the subtlest of changes in them. There are wide individual differences, and features present from childhood or puberty are generally unimportant; only recent changes are cause for concern.

Conduct the visual phase of the examination before a mirror, preferably lighted from the side, looking for alterations in the shape of the breast and nipple and in the texture of the skin. You must inspect the breasts from several positions in order to detect tumors embedded near the chest. In the tactile phase, performed once while standing and repeated while lying down, check for unusual nipple secretions and probe the spongelike tissues of the breasts for lumps.

Discovery of a lump should not be alarming; 60 to 80 per cent turn out to be harmless. But any sudden change in the breast—visual or tactile—should be reported immediately to a physician. In the unlikely event that the change indicates a malignancy, a delay of even a few weeks in reporting the symptom can result in much more difficult and extensive treatment, because breast cancer spreads rapidly, sometimes doubling in size in four weeks.

What to look for—and where

NIPPLE DIRECTION
A nipple that changes direction—suddenly pointing inward instead of projecting, or markedly shifting its angle of projection—may signal an embedded tumor.

NIPPLE SECRETIONS
Liquid that oozes from just one small part of a nipple rather than the entire nipple area, particularly if the nipple is not squeezed, can indicate a tumor.

AREOLA SIZE
Any noticeable variation, such as puckering or swelling, from past appearance of the dark halo—or areola—that surrounds each nipple is a warning signal.

UNDERARM LUMPS
Soft lumps, common and harmless under the arms of overweight women, should be checked regularly and closely for changes in size or shape.

THICKENED TISSUE
Bands of thick, fibrous tissue that can be felt in the upper parts of heavy breasts and in the "shelving margin" underneath are a concern if they suddenly change in size.

BULGE
A surface bulge, most often in the quarter of the breast nearest the armpit but sometimes elsewhere, may be external evidence of a tumor.

"ORANGE PEEL" SKIN
An unusual enlargement of pores, roughening skin texture anywhere on the breast, can be caused by a tumor that blocks channels carrying the fluid called lymph.

DIMPLES
If the previously convex contour of the breast becomes concave at any point, developing a dimple, the depression may indicate the pull of a tumor.

INTERNAL LUMPS
Most breast lumps are harmless—but new ones, particularly if hard and immovable, or old ones that grow, require a physician's attention.

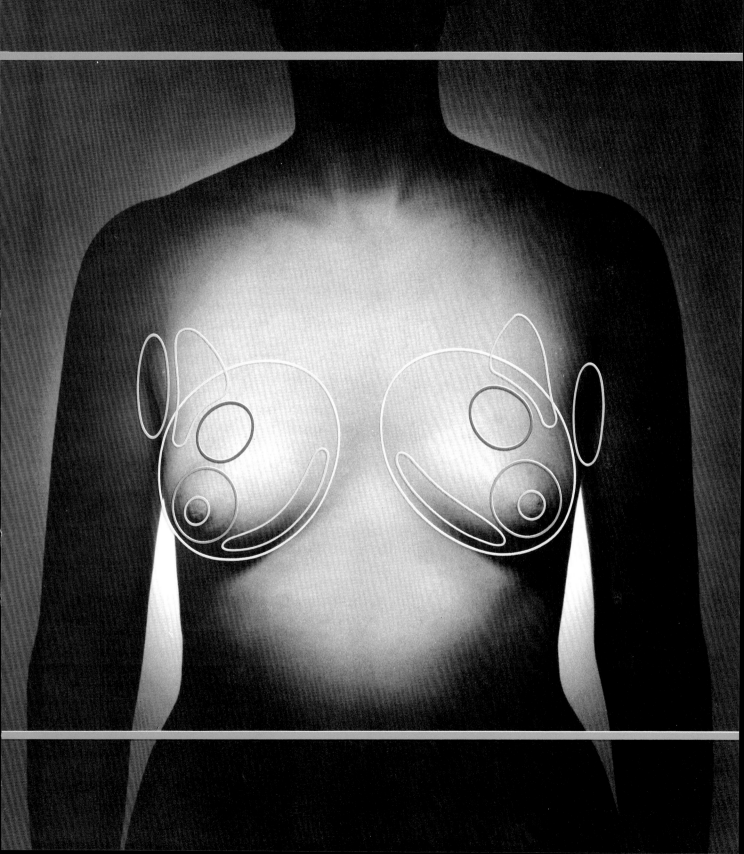

Signs that can be seen

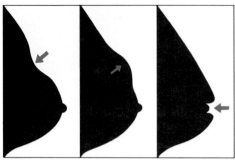

Arrows point to changes to observe in breast appearance: a dimple (left), a bulge (center) and an inverted nipple (right). Only a change is important; the conditions are common and, if long standing, are harmless.

BENDING FORWARD
With hands held at the waist, behind the back or forward on a chair, lean forward. Study the breasts to learn what is normal; in later examinations, look for changes like those sketched above. Report even a slight change immediately to a physician.

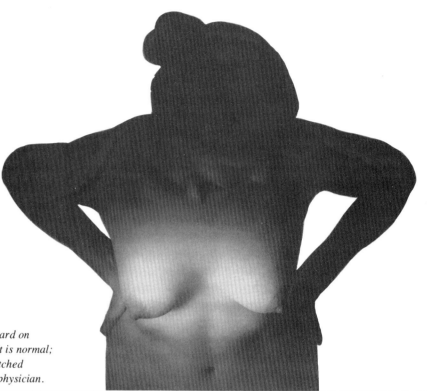

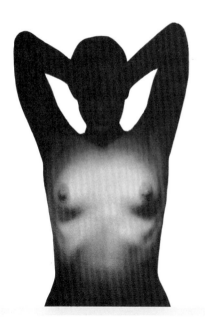

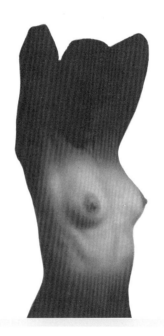

HANDS BEHIND HEAD
Continue the examination by clasping hands behind the head and pushing elbows back to stretch the skin of the breasts. Slowly rotate the upper body from side to side and look for dimples or bulges, especially on the undersides of the breasts.

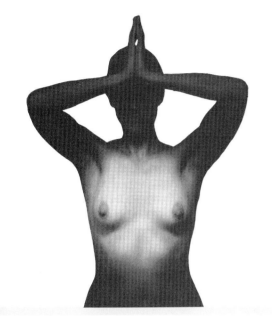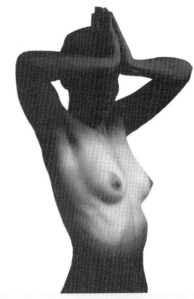

HANDS TO FOREHEAD

Press the palms of the hands firmly together in front of the forehead and rotate the upper body from side to side while looking for otherwise hidden dimples and distortions. Dimples that appear on both breasts and that are equal in size and shape are usually harmless.

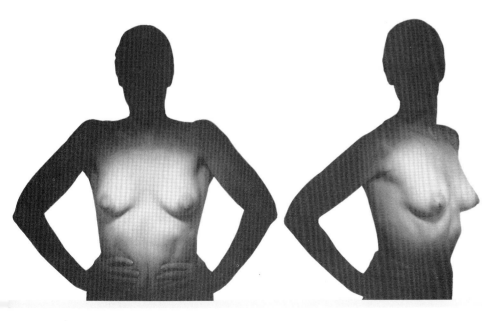

HANDS ON HIPS

Complete the visual examination by firmly pressing hands downward on the hips while holding the shoulders back. Rotate the body slowly from side to side, checking for new bulges, dimples or any other changes in appearance.

Clues that can be felt

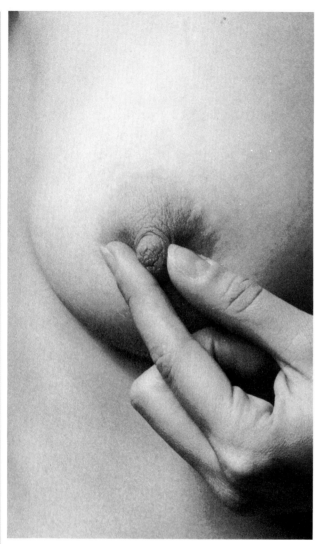

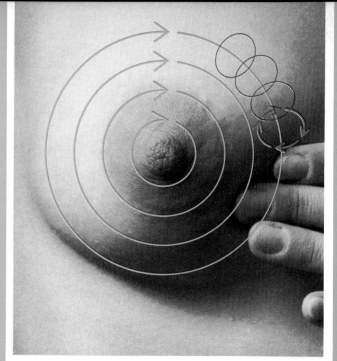

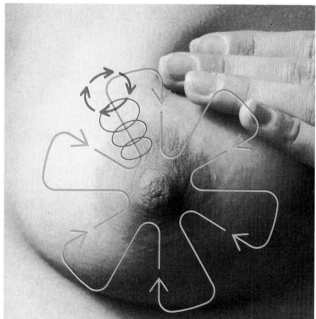

CHECKING NIPPLE SECRETIONS

*Begin the tactile examination by gently pinching each nipple.
If some secretion is released without forceful squeezing and flows
from a single pore in one breast, it may be a danger sign.
However, white, yellow, brown or even bloody secretions are
not uncommon, especially during or after a pregnancy;
they are generally harmless if they flow from many pores in both
nipples and occur only when the nipples are squeezed.*

CHECKING FOR LUMPS: STANDING

*Stand under a shower and lather the breasts, then place the left
arm at the back of the neck. Set the flat area of the finger tips
of the right hand on the rim of the left breast, directly above the
nipple, and roll the skin over the underlying tissue in small,
circular movements (red), feeling for lumps or thickenings. For
small or average-sized breasts (top), continue the movements
in at least three clockwise circles (blue), each an inch closer to the
nipple. Repeat the procedure with the opposite breast and
hand. For large breasts (bottom), make small circular movements
with the fingers down from the top-center, or 12 o'clock
position, to the nipple. Repeat these circular movements out
toward 1 o'clock, over to 2 o'clock, and so on.*

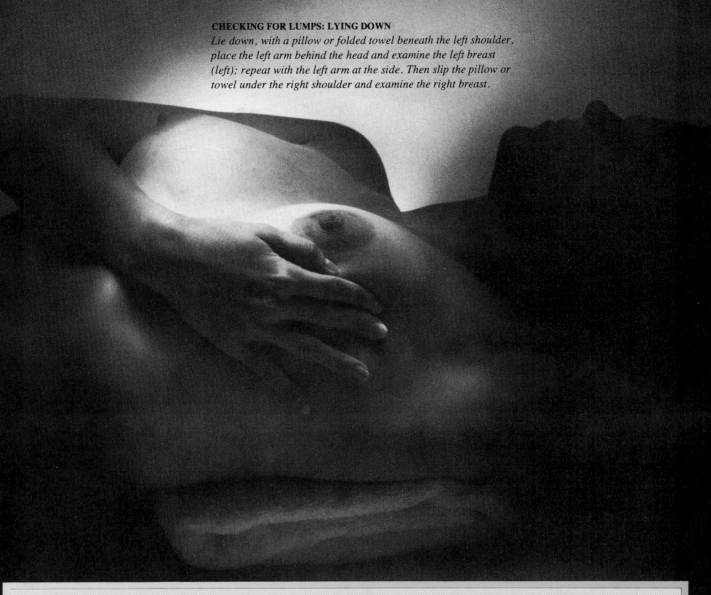

Lumps: mostly harmless, occasionally dangerous

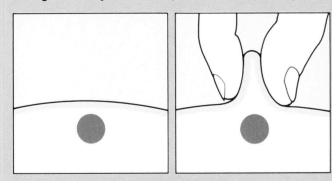

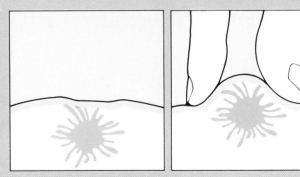

SMOOTH, SLIPPERY AND INCONSEQUENTIAL
Harmless lumps in the breast, such as milk glands, fat lobules and benign cysts, are usually smooth and movable. Pinching the skin over such a lump (above, right) generally lifts the skin away. But deciding which lumps should be examined further is a task for a physician, who seldom relies on tactile examinations alone.

ROUGH, HARD AND WORRISOME
Cancer reaches out like a crab, embedding itself within the breast tissue; a malignant tumor lies hard and fixed under the skin and feels rough, like a cocklebur (above, left). When pinched, the skin will not lift away from the lump (above, right). Many fixed lumps are not cancer, but any should be examined by a doctor.

CHAPTER 3

Unmasking the enemy

A process of elimination
The basic tests
Seeing inside by sound and heat
X-rays: new refinements of an old tool
Tracing tumors with hot atoms
The answer in a tissue sample

The heartening victories over cancer are due in large measure to new methods of treatment — but also to tremendous advances in diagnosis. Today, thanks to an arsenal of modern technologies, doctors can detect malignancies early enough to win the battle.

Long tubes of glass fibers thread television lenses through body passages to give views of tissues deep inside the lungs, stomach and other organs. Computerized X-rays create composite pictures in color and even in three dimensions. Other machines bounce sound waves off internal organs and, by measuring their echo patterns, locate tumors. Still others reveal, in glowing color images, the different heat patterns emitted by cancerous and normal tissue. Even blood tests, an old diagnostic stand-by, are being used in new ways to find circulating substances that a few years ago were not even known, much less associated with cancer.

But all the chemistry and electronics of the medical laboratory are of little use if the patient himself fails to notice the first sign that something in his body is not quite right. It may be a tinge of blood in the stool, a hacking cough that persists and worsens or a little lump that a woman had never before noticed in her breast.

This early awareness of something wrong begins the process of diagnosis. The case of Rose Kushner is typical and informative.

Dusk was settling over the Washington suburb where Rose Kushner lived, as she drew a bath, slipped into the water and leaned back for a moment, anticipating the eve-

ning's television fare. Then she began shaving under her arms. As she slid the razor under her left arm, her little finger brushed over something irregular — a tiny bump on the edge of her left nipple.

"There's something hard there," she thought, then told herself, "maybe it's nothing." But Rose Kushner was a medical writer by profession and she knew all too well what the sudden appearance of a breast lump could mean.

Frozen with fear, she remained in the bathtub for what seemed like hours. Finally her husband opened the bathroom door. "What's keeping you? Dinner is — " He stopped mid-sentence, reading something strange in her expression.

The rest of the weekend was a blur. In her book, *Breast Cancer,* Rose Kushner, who was to become a prominent spokeswoman for victims of the disease, described the time between finding the lump and seeing her doctor as "hours of bizarre charades. I tried to read *The Washington Post,* cooked breakfast, and even had friends over for an early summer barbecue." But it was "all done automatically," like sleepwalking.

By 8:30 Monday morning Mrs. Kushner was in her car, nervously driving to her internist, Dr. Bernard Heckman. The preliminary stages of diagnosis began as soon as she sat down in an examining room and Dr. Heckman began to question her. Flipping through her chart, he asked, "You've never had lumps before, have you?"

The first piece of the diagnostic puzzle was about to be put in place. A history of breast lumps — variously called fibro-

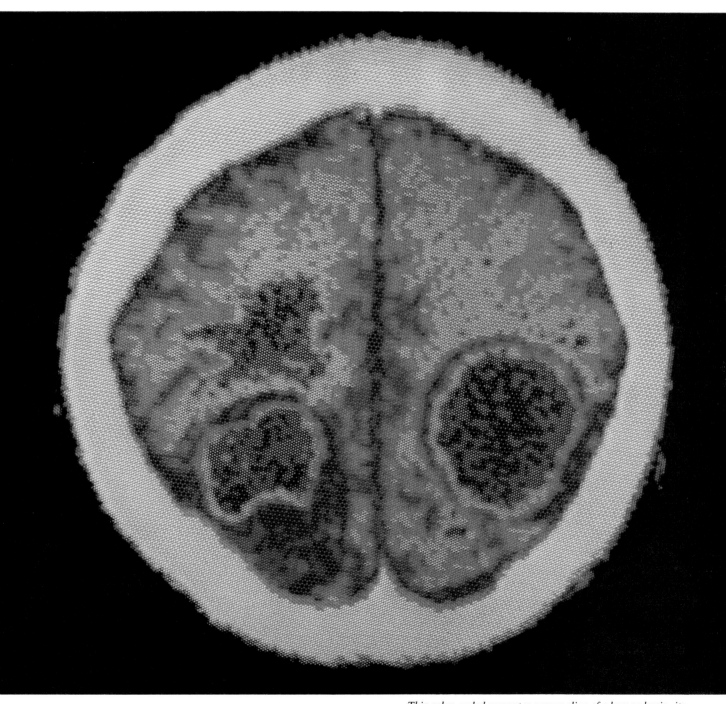

This color-coded computer-screen slice of a human brain, its green areas indicating possible tumors, was made by a CAT (for "computerized axial tomography") scanner, hailed as the most significant advance in diagnosis since the discovery of X-rays. Its pulsing X-ray source rotates around the patient, allowing a computer to construct a cross-sectional image.

cystic breasts, cystic mastitis or benign breast tumors — predisposes a woman to breast cancer, some doctors believe. But Dr. Heckman was aware that this patient had never had any problems with such lumps.

Next, Dr. Heckman asked if there had been any breast cancer in her immediate family. Breast cancer in a woman's mother or sisters also seems to increase the likelihood of cancer, possibly because of some unknown genetic factor. No one in Rose Kushner's family had ever been a victim of cancer of the breast.

Dr. Heckman, as the Kushner family doctor, knew that other conditions linked with breast cancer — no children or a first born after the age of 30 — did not apply. Rose Kushner had three teen-age sons, born when she was in her twenties. But she had begun to menstruate early, at the age of 10, and she was Jewish, two factors that are generally accepted as increasing a woman's risks for breast cancer.

Dr. Heckman's next step was to examine the lump itself. He looked at the skin covering the lump for redness, swelling, any slight depressions or "dimples," and he checked whether the nipple was drawn back, or "retracted." Any of these signs would suggest the presence of breast cancer. He found none of them.

Next the doctor carefully felt the patient's breasts. He pressed his finger tips gently in small circles around the perimeter and then moved them toward the center, feeling for the lump. He was trying to determine whether the lump was movable or stationary, whether it had distinct or spidery edges and whether it was hard or soft. Lumps that are soft, movable and contained are usually noncancerous or cancers in an early stage. More advanced malignancies tend to be hard, stationary lumps with irregular borders.

Next, Dr. Heckman reached under his patient's arms to feel the lymph nodes, tiny glands that fight disease and often harbor cancer cells. Breast cancer, if not checked early, almost always spreads to the nearby lymph nodes, and from there it can go on through the vessels of the lymph system to other parts of the body.

Dr. Heckman found no other lumps. The one Rose Kushner had detected, however, in the left breast, felt hard. Somewhat alarmed, he began a closer examination of the breast.

"Let's try to get some light on the subject," said Dr. Heckman, attempting to break the tension as he turned off the room lights and flashed a powerful focused beam on the lump. Transillumination, as the light test is called, shows a noncancerous lump — often a fluid-filled cyst — as a light shadow. A cancer, because it is more solid, appears darker, sometimes almost black.

"It looks pretty solid to me," the physician said. "I'd like you to have a mammogram," referring to an X-ray of the breast, one of the many tests that Rose Kushner was to undergo before her breast cancer was definitely diagnosed and safely removed.

A process of elimination

With his preliminary questioning in that first examination for breast cancer, Mrs. Kushner's doctor had begun the medical sleuthing procedure called differential diagnosis. It is simply a process of elimination by which physicians weed out the myriad possible ailments that could be responsible for a patient's symptoms.

Whether the patient comes to the doctor's office with a complaint as specific as a lump or as vague as abdominal discomfort, the doctor will usually begin with some general queries about past illnesses, and ailments that run in the family. The doctor may already have this medical history from past visits, but he will review it.

In addition, he will ask about — or update — details on everyday life such as smoking, drinking, diet, work environment, age of sexual maturity and level of sexual activity. These questions may seem irrelevant to the patient worried about a symptom. But an obscure and seemingly unimportant fact often turns out to be a key piece in helping to solve the diagnostic puzzle.

The painstaking step-by-step process of differential diagnosis is necessary because the symptom that sends a patient to a physician is generally typical of dozens of quite different ailments. Some are inconsequential and others are as serious as cancer.

Blood in the stool, for example, can be caused by hemorrhoids, cirrhosis of the liver, a vitamin K deficiency, stomach irritation, a peptic ulcer or an intestinal obstruction. Another cause could be stomach cancer. If abdominal pain is present as well, the doctor can probably rule out hemorrhoids, cirrhosis and the vitamin deficiency.

The doctor is then left with four possibilities: stomach irritation, a peptic ulcer, an intestinal obstruction or stomach cancer. To distinguish among them, the questions and probings of an office examination are generally inadequate, and more elaborate laboratory tests become necessary.

When a 14-year-old boy complained of fatigue and came down with a fever and cough, his doctor diagnosed a viral infection. But after 10 days of medication, the boy's condition was no better; in fact, breathing became increasingly difficult. Because the youth had suffered from asthma, he was next treated for that ailment. After a month, still no better, he was admitted to the hospital for several days of testing. At one point because of the severity of his illness, his heart stopped and he had to be revived.

The tests proved fruitful, for a chest X-ray revealed fluid on both sides of his chest as well as around his heart. The chest abnormalities were traced to a tumorous thymus gland; he had a cancer of the lymph system that could be treated with chemotherapy and radiation.

The symptoms of eight-year-old Babe Canuso also mystified her doctors for some time. The New Jersey girl had fallen while ice-skating and soon afterward began complaining of pains in her arms and legs. X-rays showed no broken bones. Babe, however, kept saying her arms and legs ached, and she grew increasingly irritable and tired. Finally her doctor ordered a blood test, and it revealed the abnormal abundance of white blood cells that signals acute lymphocytic leukemia, a type of cancer that now, in most cases, is curable in children, with the help of drugs.

The basic tests

These two children had different types of cancer, and the tests that ultimately established their diagnoses were different. Yet the differences are mainly matters of detail. Almost all cancer patients, whatever the final result of the differential

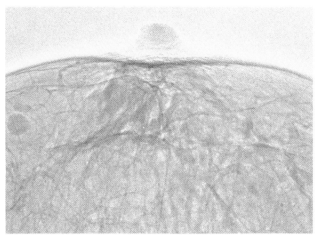

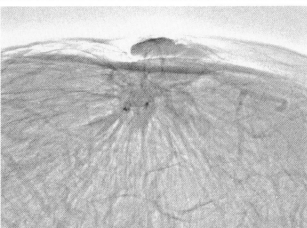

How breast X-rays called mammograms reveal cancer is seen in these pictures. At top, the uniform density of tissue and a normally projecting nipple are signs of a healthy breast. At bottom, the dense, dark mass suggests malignancy by its prickly, spreading tentacles, which pull the nipple abnormally inward—a symptom that is often the first warning (pages 64-69).

diagnosis process, go through a series of tests that are fundamentally similar. In every case, the patient is given a blood test to find out what substances are flowing through the body and in what amounts; urine tests are done to check on what and how much is being excreted. For all but a few types of cancer, some device is used to look inside the body for tumors. The looking may be done using any of dozens of kinds of X-ray machines, a tube with an eyepiece or a television camera or perhaps a scanner that generates images from radioactivity, heat or sound echoes.

The final test for cancer is always a biopsy—the removal of some cells from the patient's body for examination with a microscope to see if any are malignant. The biopsy cells may be collected simply from blood or sputum or from a swab of a body cavity, or they may have to be obtained from a surgical incision in an area under suspicion.

All these diagnostic tests are usually put into two categories: noninvasive and invasive. Those procedures that require anesthesia for the patient's comfort are considered invasive—something painful must be done to the body. Often the patient undergoing invasive tests will need to stay in the hospital overnight.

Among the noninvasive tests the most common are blood and urine analyses. Requiring at most only the prick of a needle, they may be done for many reasons: to check levels of normal blood substances or to look for abnormal substances associated with a variety of illnesses and with certain cancers. Such blood tests often reveal the abnormal white cells that signal leukemia.

More complex blood-sample analyses detect chemicals that can warn of oncoming cancers even before any symptoms are apparent. For example, CEA (for carcinoembryonic antigen) and AFP (alpha-fetoprotein) seem to be present in the blood of many people who have certain cancers. CEA, a protein on the surface of cells that have not matured properly, is presumed to be shed from cancers of the colon and rectum. The protein AFP normally exists on fetal cells, but it sometimes shows up on cancer cells too, often in cancer of the liver. With further refinement, techniques for analyzing these chemicals and other body substances eventually may

Which tests to take—and when

To discover signs of cancer at its earliest, most treatable stages, a number of simple medical examinations taken at regular intervals are recommended by cancer specialists the world over. The list at right, adapted from recommendations of the American Cancer Society for people who have no symptoms of illness, is generally accepted as authoritative in the United States.

The recommendations for tests that are considered advisable change over the years. Until 1980, for example, annual chest X-rays to spot lung cancer were urged for heavy smokers. But in 1980, the society reversed itself, contending that X-rays, which can be harmful, cannot detect lung cancer early enough to serve a useful purpose. Similarly, the recommendation for an annual Pap smear, which detects cervical cancer, was changed. A test every three years is now thought to preserve "most of the effectiveness of annual screening" at much less cost.

Expense influences many recommendations. For example, sigmoidoscopy, which offers a thorough check for tumors of the colon and rectum, is considered too costly by Italy's Istituto Nazionale per lo Studio e la Cura dei Tumori to be used unless other symptoms arouse suspicions of disease. In the United States, on the other hand, it is recommended as a routine step in regular examinations of men and women older than 50.

become accurate and painless ways of predicting cancer.

As simple—for the patient at least—as blood and urine tests are those that collect sloughed-off cells from the body for microscopic examination. One such procedure is the Pap test *(pages 78-79)*, a swab of a woman's cervix to obtain cells, which are then examined microscopically to determine the presence of cancer. Another uses sputum, the material coughed up from the lungs, to detect lung cancer. The patient breathes salt-water mist through a tube, and the mist induces

THE PART OF THE BODY EXAMINED	THE TEST	WHO SHOULD HAVE THE TEST	HOW OFTEN THE TEST IS NEEDED
Thyroid gland **Testicles and prostate gland of men** **Ovaries of women** **Mouth and skin** **Lymph nodes in the neck and pelvis and under the arms**	GENERAL CHECK UP: Visual and tactile examination by physician	Men and women over 20	Every three years until age 40 and each year thereafter
Colon and Rectum	STOOL-SLIDE TEST: Sample is placed on treated paper that detects hidden blood.	Men and women over 50	Each year
	DIGITAL RECTAL EXAM: Physician probes manually for abnormalities.	Men and women over 40	Each year
	SIGMOIDOSCOPY: Physician inserts an illuminated tube in the rectum and looks for abnormal growths.	Men and women over 50	Each year for two years: if both are negative every three to five years thereafter
Cervix	PAP SMEAR: Physician swabs cells off the cervix for examination under a microscope.	Women aged 20 to 65; also women younger than 20 who are sexually active	Each year for two years; if both are negative, every three years thereafter
Uterus	PELVIC EXAMINATION: Visual and tactile check of genital tract	Women over 20	Every three years until age 40 and each year thereafter
	ENDOMETRIAL TISSUE SAMPLE: Cells scraped from the mucous membrane that lines the uterus for examination under a microscope	Women nearing menopause	Once
Breast	BREAST SELF-EXAMINATION: (see photographs on pages 64-69)	Women over 20	Each month
	BREAST EXAMINATION BY PHYSICIAN OR NURSE	Women over 20	Every three years until age 40 and each year thereafter
	MAMMOGRAM: An x-ray of the breast	Women over 35	Once before age 40; from age 40 to age 50, only on physician's advice; over age 50, each year

him to cough and expel sputum into a jar. The cells in the sputum can reveal a lung cancer that is still too small to show up on a chest X-ray.

Seeing inside by sound and heat

Most of the methods for viewing the inside of the body are similarly painless and noninvasive. Two new techniques coming into wide use depend on sound or heat waves to create images similar to X-ray pictures.

The sonic method is called ultrasound because it employs tones too high-pitched to be heard. It is occasionally used to detect breast lumps, but is most valuable when looking for tumors deep in the body—in the pancreas, kidney, ovaries or endometrium, the lining of the womb.

To check for possible endometrial cancer, one typical patient, a 49-year-old Minneapolis secretary, had an ultrasound test. As she lay on an examining table, a technician swabbed mineral oil on her abdomen; the oil helps conduct sound waves and keeps outside noise from being picked up by the microphone-like probe that is pressed to the abdomen. The only sensation this patient recalled was the cool touch of the plastic probe moving silently across her midsection. The probe beamed in the sound waves, then it picked up the echoes bouncing off her body organs. These reflected sounds—translated into dotted patterns that look like weather maps—were displayed on a television monitor. The test was completed in half an hour, and three days later the results were in: The woman did indeed have endometrial cancer—but in a form easily cured by simple surgery.

Ultrasound can be used to distinguish between solid tumors and fluid-filled cysts—because liquids make echo patterns different from those of firm areas—but the technique will not prove whether a solid area is cancerous. The difference between cancerous and noncancerous tissue can be recorded, however, by a heat test called thermography, which measures the distinctive heat patterns that body tissues, including tumors, give off. Some thermographic devices are massive units that look like X-ray machines; others are experimental gadgets so small that they are worn inside a brassiere for detecting breast lumps.

One thermography technique, called graphic stress telethermometry, or GST, tests for cancer by stressing the body with sudden, intense cold. Benign lumps will cool off during the test, but cancerous tumors remain hot because circulation in them is so poor that heat is less readily dissipated.

"The worst part of it was the frigid room temperature," recalled Peggy Matthews, a 32-year-old New York writer who underwent a GST of suspicious breast lumps. The examining room is kept at 63° F. so that the sensor will pick up only body heat and not be influenced by the temperature of surroundings. A detecting wand, not unlike the microphone-probe in ultrasound, was first passed over Peggy Matthews' breasts—without touching them—to measure their pattern of heat emissions.

Then came the stress. Peggy Matthews remembers, "I had to plunge my hands into a plastic basin filled with ice water and ice cubes for 15 seconds, which felt like an eternity." After she removed her hands from the freezing water,

the detecting wand was passed over her breasts again.

A few days later Peggy Matthews got the results. The GST indicated noncancerous cysts, confirming an earlier X-ray—when both thermography and an X-ray show the same results for a breast lump, accuracy of the paired diagnostic procedures rises to 95 per cent.

X-rays: new refinements of an old tool

The X-ray may well be the most familiar of all the diagnostic tests used to locate tumors. In the same painless way that an X-ray reveals a dental cavity or a broken bone, it can pinpoint a tumor. In the basic type of X-ray, almost universally employed to detect lung, breast and bone tumors, low-level radiation passes through tissue onto a sensitized film, and the resulting shadow picture shows differences in tissue density. Malignant lumps, which are denser than noncancerous lumps or normal tissue, are more pronounced on film.

The likelihood of discovering cancer with this basic type of X-ray increases if the tumor is relatively large and is denser than the surrounding area or if it is located in soft tissue in the outer area of an organ. Others may escape detection. A pea-sized cancer that is growing in a major airway deep within the lungs, for example, will probably be more difficult to find than another many times smaller that is located on the edge of a lung.

The difficulty of X-raying small tumors surrounded by a good deal of normal tissue led to the development of a special type of X-ray, called a mammogram, now routinely used for breast examination. The breast is so much thicker toward the chest than at the nipple that, for ordinary X-rays, varying amounts of radiation are needed to make a clear picture. The mammogram avoids this problem by X-raying the breast while it is compressed slightly to equalize its thickness.

Some women find that although the mammogram procedure is painless it can be uncomfortable. Betty Rollin, a television news correspondent who was successfully treated for breast cancer, described her first mammogram this way: "Holding your paper gown together with one hand and grabbing your purse, bra and blouse with the other, you are bustled off to a room where, topless and chilly, you sit on a small

Technicians monitor a CAT scanner as it simulates the creation
of a cross-sectional image of a model's head. In practice, the CAT
scanner shoots hundreds of X-rays through the brain from
every angle. Detectors pick up the X-rays and a computer displays
them on monitor screens—in black and white (bottom left),
color (page 71) or simulated three dimensions (bottom right).

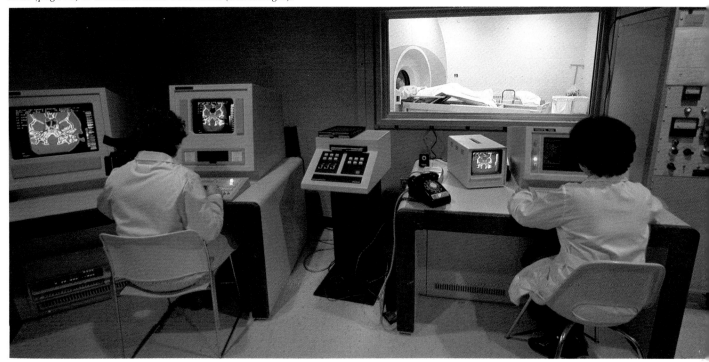

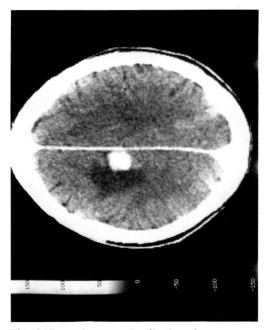

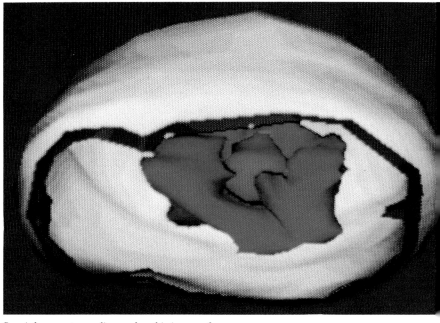

This CAT scan image, a visualization of
variations in tissue density, reveals a tumor
below the membrane between the brain's
two hemispheres. By assigning colors
to the densities, the computer can convert
a black-and-white picture to color.

Special computer coding makes this image of
a brain CAT scan show not only color but
also three dimensions, greatly simplifying
the task of locating the tumor (red)
and the surrounding distended tissue (blue)
within the patient's skull (yellow).

stool before a large machine. A technician takes your breast in her hand and puts it, as if it were a slab of beef, on a slab of steel. She cranks down another slab of steel, thereby creating a breast sandwich. Your flattened breast is the filling.''

The discomfort is worthwhile. The mammogram images show the breast's delicate network of blood vessels, ducts and glands, muscles and fat. What also will show up—clearly visible as dark spots—are common breast cysts, blood clots, and benign or malignant tumors. One of the newer devices adapts the office copying machine to produce pictures instantly, on paper instead of film. These ''xeromammograms'' *(page 73)* are also easier for a radiologist to read because the images are blue and white instead of the shades of gray created in an X-ray or mammogram made on film.

The breast is an organ easily investigated by X-ray. Tumors in other soft but inaccessible organs such as the brain, pancreas, bladder and liver were more difficult to X-ray clearly until the advent of the specialized machine called the CAT scanner (for ''computerized axial tomography''), which won its inventors the 1979 Nobel prize. The CAT scanner *(page 77)* produces a cross-sectional view, as if a

slice were pulled out of the body and examined from all angles in much the same way a slice of bread might be lifted out of the center of a loaf.

To make such a cross section, some 100 to 200 narrow X-ray beams are sent from an arc around a section of the body, say the brain; after each beam passes through, its intensity is measured. In this way, the densities of tissue in thousands of points within the brain are measured from hundreds of different angles.

The detector then forwards this data to a computer, which assigns to each point a number indicating the amount of radiation the tissue there had absorbed. The computer translates the numbers into a color-coded screen image. In some CAT scanners further coding produces a three-dimensional image, which aids in diagnosing a tumor's size and position.

Since the introduction of the CAT scan to cancer diagnosis, a faster and more precise machine for scanning has been developed: the dynamic spatial reconstructor. It can make 75,000 cross-sectional images of the body in the time it takes the CAT scanner to make one—about five seconds. It not only can create cross-sectional slices but can also dice the

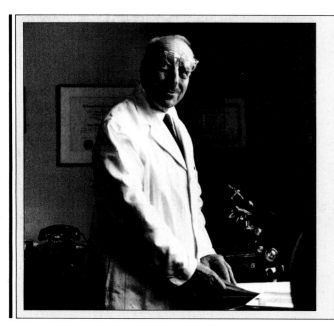

George N. Papanicolaou, Dr. Pap of the Pap smear

Dr. Pap's lifesaving smear

The Pap test, a simple and painless procedure *(drawing, right)* that has saved uncounted women's lives by detecting cancer of the cervix early enough for cure, was devised by a Greek immigrant physician, George Nicholas Papanicolaou, whose first job in America, in 1913, was selling rugs in a department store. But within a year he had a position in his professional specialty at Cornell University Medical College. There in 1925 Dr. Pap, as he came to be called, discovered that a small smear of vaginal cells could reliably indicate the presence of cancer.

Dr. Papanicolaou published his findings in 1928, but the test was not widely employed until after World War II, following his development of a staining technique that made the cell abnormalities easily visible. The Pap smear quickly became a standard part of every woman's routine physical. Before he died in 1962, Dr. Pap saw the death rate for cervical cancer cut, thanks largely to his pioneering research, by almost 50 per cent.

body—lengthwise, crosswise, diagonally or in any other way—so that the doctor can call up on a screen a three-dimensional image of any part of the patient's body. The image made by the dynamic spatial reconstructor can be shown at any angle—and in motion.

For many cancer diagnoses the clarity of X-ray pictures—whether made by simple machines or computerized scanners—can be enhanced if the patient drinks, inhales or is injected with a "contrast" chemical mixture that makes soft tissues more opaque to X-rays than they normally are. X-rays cannot pass through the contrast mixture, and the organ that has absorbed it will show up as a distinct image on the film.

Nearly every part of the body can be visualized with some form of contrast X-ray. A contrast "cocktail" containing a harmless compound of the heavy element barium may simply be swallowed—it looks like a strawberry milkshake but does not taste much like one—to reveal the contours of the esophagus, stomach or small intestines. A contrast material such as barium or a chemical dye may be administered rectally in an enema to highlight the colon, or sent through a catheter to show the bladder or uterus.

More complex contrast X-rays may involve some pain and are considered invasive tests. Dyes containing iodine may be injected into the spleen, spinal cord, heart or lungs, into the carotid artery of the neck to search out tumors of the head and neck, or into other veins and arteries to see if cancer has affected the body's blood supply.

Typical of these contrast X-ray procedures is the survey of the lymph system *(pages 106-107)* that produces a lymphangiogram. The test is usually done to trace the progress of a lymph cancer such as Hodgkin's disease. But it also is used to see whether any tumor has spread elsewhere, for the lymph system often transports malignant cells from the original cancer throughout the body.

Such a wandering cancer is what doctors were looking for when they performed a lymphangiogram on Cornelius Ryan, author of *The Longest Day* and *A Bridge Too Far,* who eventually died of prostate cancer. At the time of his lymphangiogram, his prostate tumor had already been diagnosed. The question to be answered by this test was how far malignancy had spread.

"First they shaved my feet and painted them with disinfec-

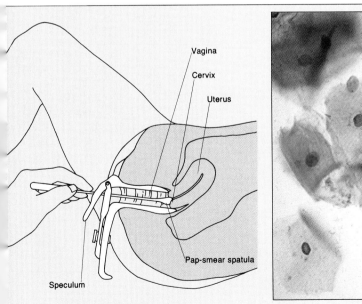
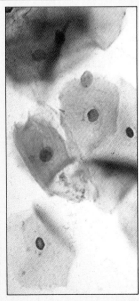
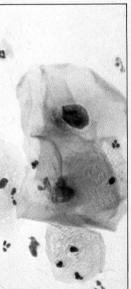
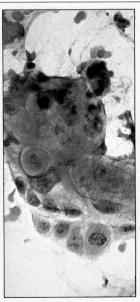

For a Pap smear the physician uses a speculum to stretch apart the vaginal walls, in the pelvis (dark purple). The cervix, at the tip of the uterus, is then swabbed for cells, which are smeared on a slide and sent to a laboratory for study.

Cells from the cervix are stained to make the central nuclei dark purple and the surrounding material, cytoplasm, blue in young cells and pink in older ones. Normal cells (above, left) have small nuclei. Larger, less regular nuclei (center) may suggest precancerous growth. At right, amid red blood cells are cancer-stricken cells, all their normal structure destroyed.

tant,'' Ryan wrote in *A Private Battle*. ''Novocain was injected and then a surgeon made an incision into the dorsal lymphatics,'' the lymph channels on the tops of the feet. The feet are generally chosen as the site of the incision because lymph fluid, unlike blood, flows in only one direction—from the body's remote tissue beds to the base of the neck, where it enters the bloodstream.

Injected into the feet is an oil-based contrast material mixed with blue dye. It moves up the body through the lymph canals, collecting in and highlighting the dozens of lymph glands, some the size of a pea, others larger than a walnut. A few hours later, once the dye has had time to reach every nook and cranny of the lymph system, X-rays are taken of the entire body. The process can take as long as five hours, start to finish.

''The time, the pain, the mounting boredom are all very hard to take,'' Ryan wrote. ''Had I not been comforted and attended to throughout that time by an expert technician, I don't know if I could have kept control.''

For a 27-year-old singer named Ruth Cullen, who underwent a lymphangiogram for the lymph-system cancer called Hodgkin's disease, the test proved equally depressing. ''There's something humiliating about it,'' she said. ''This was three hours, and they had to keep turning me over and twisting me around. I felt like a piece of meat.'' Yet she herself became an example of the procedure's value. Soon after her early diagnosis, she began a course of treatment, and within a year her disease was in a state of remission that her doctors believe may well extend to a natural life span.

Tracing tumors with hot atoms

X-rays are not the only atomic phenomena that can be exploited to make pictures of cancers that lie deep inside the body. One device that came into use in the 1970s, the focused

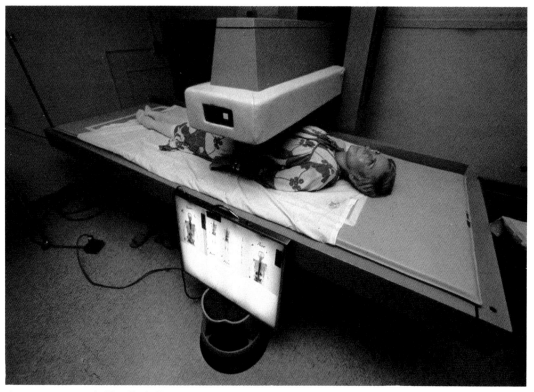

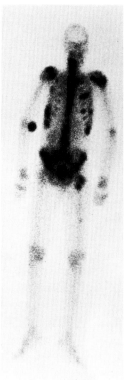

At a cancer center in New York City, a patient injected with a radioactive fluid lies beneath a bone scanner, which reveals the spread of cancer. The fluid builds up in cancerous tissue, and the scanner makes a film record of these radioactive hot spots. In the scan at right, of another patient, black areas show cancer spread to shoulders, spine, pelvis, ribs and elbow.

nuclear magnetic resonance scanner, tunes in to the magnetic radiations emitted by the body's atoms—carbon, hydrogen, oxygen and so on—as a radio tunes in to the wavelengths of specific stations to pick up broadcasts. The scanner can detect radiations that show something is wrong inside the living cell; and it can create a visual image of the trouble spot, much as a CAT scan does, but without having to process data through a computer. What is more, it can zoom in on the suspicious area and identify, from the nature of the radiations, the chemical nature of their source. In this way it helps the doctor determine whether the cause of trouble is tuberculosis, a benign cyst or cancer.

More commonly used than nuclear magnetism are the radiations of a variety of weakly radioactive materials, which are introduced into the body and accumulate in specific organs—that is, each type of material is selectively absorbed by a particular organ so that it concentrates there. Its emanations are then recorded on film, or they are picked up by an electronic scanner, somewhat like a computerized geiger counter, that produces an image on a television screen.

The radioactive substances all emit gamma rays, a kind of radiation that in the doses used causes little or no harm to living tissue. The substances carrying the radiation are rapidly excreted from the body, and in any case they lose their radioactivity very quickly—among those substances often used, iodine 123 decreases in radioactivity by half every 13 hours and technetium 99 by half every six hours.

Such tests make use of the fact that cancer cells absorb materials at rates that are different from those of normal cells. In the test, a substance needed for cell growth of a specific organ may be made radioactive or it may be combined with another radioactive material. For example, bone cells require phosphorus, so when the physician wants to check for bone tumors, the radioactive form of that element, phosphorus 32, is introduced into the patient's body. After two hours or so— enough time for the phosphorus 32 to concentrate in the bone—a scanner is placed over the bone to measure the radioactive emissions, or a camera records an image of these emissions on film.

Because malignant cells absorb more of the mixture than normal cells, cancerous areas show up as "hot spots," much as a uranium lode shows up "hot" when a geiger counter passes over it. In a variation of this technique, a "cold spot" may indicate cancer because the particular radioactive mixture is picked up by normal cells and shunned by malignant ones; thus, a cancerous area of the thyroid gland, when treated with iodine 123, shows up as a cold spot. A scan that shows a hot or cold spot, however, does not always mean cancer; for example, a bone fracture or an arthritic joint might also show up on a scan.

Most radioactivity scanners produce a flat silhouette that looks like an ordinary X-ray. A new type of scanner, called the PETT (for positron emission transaxial tomography), uses a circle of detectors to create cross-sectional images like those of a CAT scanner. But while a CAT scanner gives a picture of a patient's anatomy, the PETT scanner shows the metabolic activity of the patient's cells.

The patient is injected with a solution of a type of sugar (glucose) compounded with radioactive fluorine or oxygen so that its emissions can be detected by the scanner. In the body, healthy cells absorb the radioactive mixture at a specific rate, while cancer cells absorb it at either a slower or a faster rate.

Up to this point the preparation for a PETT scan is similar to that for an ordinary scan of radioactive tracers—but now a new technique takes over. The radioactive cells emit packets of energy called positrons, which have the peculiarity of shooting out in only two directions, exactly 180° apart. When two positron emissions hit the circle of PETT detectors at precisely the same moment, they are used for a reconstruction of the image. The computer records the source of the emissions and, like the computer of a CAT scanner, collects bits of information from many planes to show all of the organ's activity. The PETT scanner has proved particularly valuable for revealing activity within the cells of the brain.

The answer in a tissue sample

As a patient's diagnosis progresses, it is generally necessary to learn more about a suspected cancer than is possible from techniques that require only blood or urine tests, coughing,

A debate over biopsies

Many patients go into the operating room without knowing how far the surgeon will go. He must first remove small tissue samples for a biopsy—the microscopic examination that is the ultimate proof of cancer. Then, if the biopsy establishes cancer, he may schedule a later operation to remove the tumor, or he may go right ahead and remove it on the spot, without further discussion with the patient. The latter procedure—"single-stage" surgery—has aroused bitter criticism, particularly from women treated for breast cancer. They may go under anesthesia not knowing whether they will awaken with only a small incision from the biopsy—or with a breast and much chest muscle gone.

Several arguments favor the separate biopsy followed later, if necessary, by further surgery:

• The patient gets time to adjust to the idea that an important part of the body must be removed.

• Biopsy is a safe and relatively simple procedure that can be handled by any competent surgeon in a good hospital. However, for the more complex surgery that often follows, an experienced specialist working in a large cancer center may be preferable.

• The delay permits positive confirmation of the diagnosis with a "permanent-section" biopsy, which is somewhat more reliable than the "frozen-section" technique *(pages 86-91)* used for single-stage surgery.

• The patient has the opportunity to consider alternative treatments—for breast cancer the options range from the extensive surgery of the so-called radical mastectomy to non-surgical drug and radiation therapies *(Chapter 4)*.

Weighing against such arguments is the inescapable fact that, for many types of cancer, the biopsy itself requires that the body be cut open while the patient is under general anesthesia—a procedure that is traumatic and entails some risk. To many doctors and their patients, it seems preferable to get all the surgery over and done with at one time.

Thus the dispute continues. Responding to protests from patients, America's National Cancer Institute recommended in 1979 that single-stage surgery be dropped in most cases in favor of the two-stage method. However, not all surgeons and hospitals went along with the change. Among those that did not was the world-renowned Memorial Sloan-Kettering Hospital of New York City.

swabbing of easy-to-reach tissues, X-rays or radioactivity scans. The next step in diagnosis is almost always the biopsy—the removal and examination of tissues that provides the only definitive diagnosis of cancer.

Many different methods are employed to obtain the tissue for examination. When a tumor is large, a surgeon will often perform an "incisional" biopsy, cutting out a piece of the lump. When the mass is small and there is a good chance it is cancerous, he may cut out the entire lump in an "excisional" biopsy. But not all biopsies require surgical incisions. The surgeon can often obtain the tissue sample by scraping it off with brushes or tiny clippers inserted through a body opening, or by suctioning it out through a syringe, a procedure called aspiration biopsy.

Cells can be suctioned from many sites, including the breast, spinal cord, thyroid or prostate glands, or the lining of the womb. However, the procedure is used most often to remove bone marrow—the fluid and spongy tissue that manufactures blood cells in the middle of bones—to confirm a diagnosis of leukemia.

Although the patient is given a local anesthetic for a bone-marrow aspiration, the anesthetic deadens the bone less than it does the skin, so the test may be painful. If the needle is not inserted with great precision, it may also stimulate a nerve. "My legs jerked like a frog's in a laboratory experiment," wrote journalist Stewart Alsop in *Stay of Execution,* a book about his experiences with leukemia, the disease from which he eventually died.

For many types of cancers, particularly those of the breathing and digestive systems, doctors perform biopsies by inserting instruments called endoscopes down through the throat or up through the intestinal tract. There are many different types of endoscope, but all consist of some kind of tube, fitted at one end with a tiny light, a lens and brushes or clippers; at the other end are controls, an eyepiece and, in some models, a television camera. They enable the physician to look for suspicious lumps, and when he finds one, to extract some or all of it for laboratory examination.

Some endoscopes are rigid steel instruments: These include the proctosigmoidoscope, for examining the rectum and colon; the cystoscope, which is inserted under local or general anesthetic into the urethra to study the bladder; the colposcope, which is placed in the vagina to study the cervix; and the rigid bronchoscope, which checks parts of the upper respiratory tract.

Other endoscopes are long and flexible, and contain bundles of exquisitely fine glass fibers that conduct light around curves and can be looped through many feet of body passageways to investigate the darkest reaches of the body. Among these are the colonoscope, which can be threaded all the way through the six feet of the large intestine; the duodenoscope, less than half an inch wide, which can be swallowed and slid to the head of the pancreas, one of the most inaccessible body organs; and the flexible bronchoscope, which reaches inside the lungs.

When the bronchoscope, for example, is used for a lung biopsy, its brushes pick up minute samples of tissues while salt water is squirted into the lungs and retrieved by suction through a ''sidearm'' attached to the bronchoscope. Loose cells are gathered up in this ''washing'' and added to those brushed off for study.

This type of bronchoscopy is especially useful in finding lung cancer when, as often happens, an X-ray shows no indication of cancer but the simple sputum test indicates some sort of abnormality. In the case of Thomas Gregory, such a test saved his life.

''I was with the New York City Police Department, and they encouraged anyone who was 35 or older and a smoker to be checked,'' recalled Gregory, thinking back to the day when he, 55 and a heavy smoker, and a dozen of his fellow policemen went to Memorial Sloan-Kettering Cancer Center for sputum and X-ray tests. ''There was nothing on the X-ray, but right after the sputum test, I got a note saying the sputum showed abnormalities. After more sputum tests, all positive, I had my first bronchoscopy.''

That diagnostic test did not locate Gregory's cancer. But it launched him on an experience many other cancer patients have shared. For a year and a half, he underwent a variety of examinations before his tumor could be conclusively diagnosed, located and cut out.

Gregory was given the routine tests that almost every patient gets, regardless of the illness, to determine the general state of his health: an electrocardiogram, or ECG, to check the heart, and blood and urine analyses to evaluate the state of such tissues and organs as bone marrow and kidneys. For Gregory, there were also a number of tests related specifically to the lungs.

X-rays were taken of his chest. His fingers were examined for ''clubbing,'' a thickening at the tips that sometimes accompanies lung cancer. Pulmonary function tests checked breathing efficiency; these tests can tell the surgeon whether the patient will require a machine to help him breathe while on the operating table, and they indicate how well the patient's lungs will function if one or more lobes—or even an entire lung—must be removed. The lungs have five sections, or lobes—three on the right side of the body and two on the left. (The place where a third left lobe would logically be located is taken by the heart.)

In one such test of pulmonary function a soft clamp is placed on the patient's nose. He then is directed to breathe through a hose into a tank, while a meter keeps score of the flow of air in and out of his lungs. It also measures the maximum volume of air he is able to inhale.

Another test often applied, but not needed in Gregory's case, requires the patient to inhale radioactive xenon 133 gas. A scanner then counts the emissions from the tiny air sacs in the lungs to indicate how the sacs are operating.

In another test of lung function, the patient may be given an injection of radioactive technetium 99 in the arm. Cameras record how long it takes for the substance to reach the lungs, whether it is concentrated in any particular area and how it circulates through the passages. Both types of tests show whether a person's lungs trap too much or too little radioactive gas in one area so that breathing efficiency may be reduced. If not, then the lungs are functioning relatively well and do not present special hazards for a bronchoscopy.

During the year and a half of testing, Gregory underwent several bronchoscopies. The procedure is generally similar in all such tests, but his second one was the most complex.

The day of this second bronchoscopy Thomas Gregory

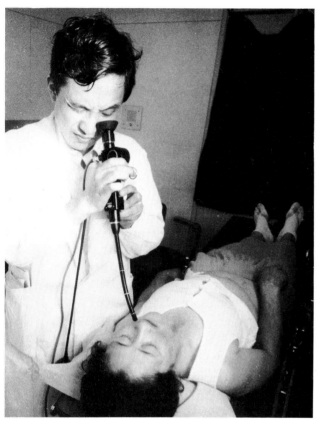

Using an endoscope, a doctor photographs the interior of a patient's stomach. The instrument contains flexible, light-transmitting fibers that can be snaked through the digestive and respiratory tracts to parts of the body once accessible only by surgery. Though mainly a diagnostic tool, an endoscope can be adapted to take tissue samples and cut out small tumors.

was given a shot of pentobarbital to make him drowsy and another of atropine to dry up body secretions. A hollow plastic tube, or catheter, was placed in his arm to be used for administering the anesthesia. He was wheeled to the operating room, where Dr. Nael Martini, Chief of Thoracic Surgery at Sloan-Kettering, waited, dressed in a sterilized scrub suit, surgical mask, hood, and sterile booties over his shoes.

Gregory lay on his back under green sterile drapes. His right arm was taped to an armboard, palm up, fingers in a grip. The catheter was hooked up to the anesthesia machine. At Dr. Martini's signal, the anesthesiologist allowed thiopental, an anesthetic, to flow through the catheter, and Gregory was soon unconscious. An oxygen mask was placed over his mouth briefly to assist his breathing.

The head of the operating table was lowered from its horizontal position to ease the delicate procedure and improve Dr. Martini's view into Gregory's throat. Dr. Martini slowly began to thread the first bronchoscope, a rigid one about a third of an inch in diameter, through Gregory's mouth and down his throat. The surgeon looked at the vocal cords—they were fine. He slid the instrument through the widest opening between the cords to the trachea, or windpipe, which is the passage for the air from larynx to lungs. Then the doctor moved the scope into the left lung's upper lobe.

A few drops of salt water were injected through the side-arm on the instrument and suctioned back up. The sample was labeled ''Thomas Gregory 57-14-21 left bronchial washing'' and sent to the pathology laboratory to be studied under a microscope. The same thing was done at the opening of each of the other lobes. Then, moving as if in slow motion, Dr. Martini removed the rigid scope, and the anesthesiologist replaced the oxygen mask.

The rigid bronchoscope gives a view of only about 20 per cent of the lungs but it can give a very clear view of that part and is used in cases such as Thomas Gregory's, where disease is difficult to locate because it is in the earliest stages. To examine the rest, Dr. Martini switched to a slender, flexible fiber-optic bronchoscope, which does not provide quite so clear an image but covers more of the lungs.

He deftly slid the flexible instrument into the windpipe,

beginning a stage that would take almost two hours. Each lung has 18 major segments and, depending on the individual, between 36 and 54 subsegments. Dr. Martini examined each one and took washings and brushings from any suspicious areas. As in the earlier bronchoscopy, the results were negative. There were no malignant tissues to prove that Gregory had cancer.

Still, the sputum tests had been positive. With Thomas Gregory's life at stake, the doctor scheduled a third bronchoscopy. This time he used the flexible fiber-optic model alone—he was sure the trouble, if any, lay deep in the lobes.

Once again he searched for more than an hour, and found nothing but normal tissue. Then at last Dr. Martini spotted a suspicious dot. There the normally pinkish mucous lining of the upper lobe of the left lung gave way to a grayish-white area. Its color suggested malignancy.

Now the surgeon slipped the tiny bronchoscopic brush into the scope's sidearm and on down to the grayish-white spot. The small bits of tissue that adhered were put on a slide and sent to the lab. More examining, more brushing and washing, and about 45 minutes later, the procedure was completed. The bronchoscope was removed, anesthesia was stopped, and mouth and throat secretions were suctioned out. Soon Gregory was transferred to a stretcher and wheeled to the recovery room.

Dr. Martini was certain he had seen malignancy, and the pathologists confirmed his judgment with a so-called permanent-section biopsy. Over several days of complicated laboratory work, the tissue sample was dipped in paraffin and put through elaborate staining procedures. The result was a slide that, viewed under the microscope, clearly revealed the presence of malignant cells.

Now a surgical operation was scheduled for Thomas Gregory. It would remove the cancerous area—and the tissue would be sent out for yet another biopsy. For this ultimate biopsy, samples would be taken not with bronchoscope brushes but with a scalpel—used to make an incision in Gregory's chest. These samples would serve to confirm the bronchoscopy diagnoses, but they would also show whether cancer had spread beyond the area indicated by bronchoscopy—information the surgeon would need to decide whether he must excise more tissue than originally planned.

About a week after the last bronchoscopy had indicated cancer—a delay that was needed to build the strength of Gregory's heart—he was once again wheeled to the operating room, semidrowsy with pentobarbital. Catheters were placed in his arms to deliver vital fluids, and probes monitored his temperature and blood pressure. Once he was unconscious, his chest was opened, the blood vessels clamped, muscles severed and the ribs spread some eight inches apart by a large steel retractor.

Dr. Martini cut away the cancerous lobe, removing the grayish tissue that the bronchoscopies had located, as well as some surrounding tissue. Then, grasping with forceps the spongy mass of tissue he had been cutting, Dr. Martini lifted it free of the chest and dropped it in a sterile pan, which was wrapped, labeled and rushed to the pathology laboratory. Other bits of tissue from lymph nodes near the lung were also packaged and sent.

In the laboratory a "frozen-section" biopsy *(pages 86-91)*—somewhat less reliable than the permanent-section type but much faster—was made. The quicker method was used this time in Gregory's case, because the suspicious area had already been located and abnormal tissue had been confirmed in previous biopsies.

There was no mistaking the cancer. Under the microscope the cells excised from Gregory's lung were crowded together unnaturally; they were irregularly shaped and their nuclei were enlarged.

One of the pathologists called the operating room. "Dr. Martini, on Thomas Gregory, patient number 57-14-21, this is an epidermoid carcinoma by previous diagnoses confirmed by frozen section." Then he gave the heartening verdict that Dr. Martini had hoped for. "The margins are clear of tumor. The lymph nodes are negative."

The last diagnosis showed no spread of cancer. Thomas Gregory's incision was closed and five years later, after repeated follow-up examinations found no recurrence, he became an encouraging statistic: one of the constantly growing number of people who have been cured of cancer. ✳

The final word: a biopsy

No matter how many tests implicate cancer, the proof that a suspicious lump is malignant must wait for a biopsy: scrutiny under a microscope of a tiny piece of the tumor tissue. The tissue sample is cut out by a surgeon. However, the crucial decision on whether or not the sample indicates malignancy is made independently by a specialist scientist known as a pathologist, who must be familiar with the normal appearance of every kind of tissue and cell in the body. If any cell or bit of tissue looks irregular, the pathologist must be prepared to explain why. The pathologist's verdict—benign or malignant—is the last word.

A detailed ''permanent section'' biopsy may require two days, but often the pathologist must render his judgment under a tight deadline, with a type of biopsy called frozen section. The tumor sample removed from the patient is flash-frozen into a solid block that can be sliced so thin that a section becomes transparent, revealing the structures of its cells to the microscope. In this sliver of tissue, the pathologist searches for cancer's telltale wreckage: cell nuclei that are enlarged or discolored, cells growing far beyond their usual numbers, or bits of tumors in lymph or blood vessels, through which cancerous cells may be traveling to set up colonies in other parts of the body.

All these steps may be completed in 15 minutes by the staff of an efficient pathology laboratory, such as that at Georgetown University Hospital in Washington, D.C., where the photographs on this and the following pages were made from the biopsies of several patients. Some 1,200 frozen sections are performed annually at Georgetown; such experience makes it possible for pathologists and surgeons to diagnose cancer and remove it in one operation—while the patient remains under anesthesia—avoiding the need for a second bout of surgery.

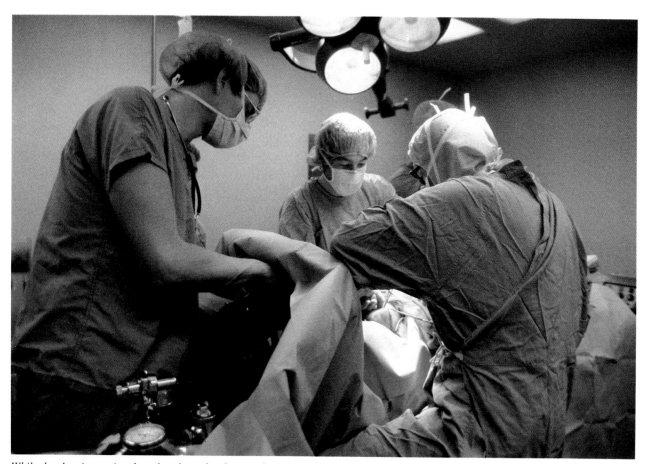

While the sleeping patient breathes through a face mask handled by an anesthesiologist (left), her surgeon (right) makes an incision to remove a small section from a part of her breast where a suspicious lump has been found. As one of the precautions that help keep the area of the operation free of infection, the patient's head is kept behind a partition of blue paper.

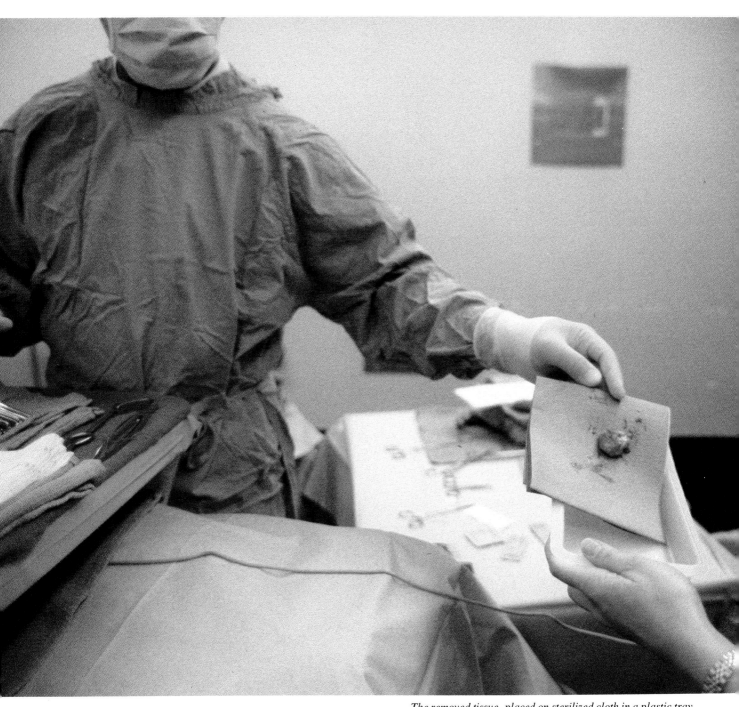

The removed tissue, placed on sterilized cloth in a plastic tray, is handed to the operating-room nurse, who carries it to the surgical-pathology laboratory just down the corridor. During the next quarter of an hour, while pathologists are examining the tissue, the surgical team stays at work, probing the area around the tumor for any signs of spreading cancer.

In the laboratory, a pathologist uses a scalpel (right) to cut off bits of tissue for a frozen-section examination. One of the fragments is set into a plastic box (below), where it stays during the freezing process. The remainder of the biopsy tissue is preserved in a formaldehyde solution for additional tests.

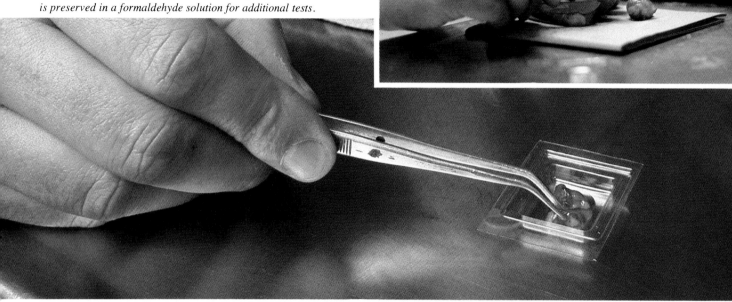

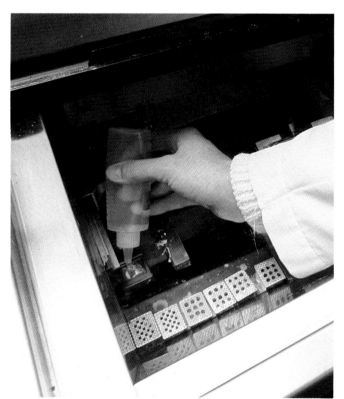

Reaching into the freezer, which reduces temperature to about −22° F. when its lid is shut, a technician fills the plastic box with a solution of alcohol and resins. A gold-colored clip (foreground) is then placed on top for use as a grip later.

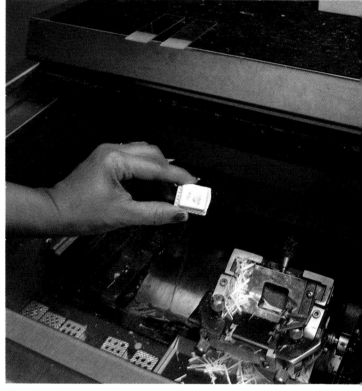

After five minutes in the freezer, the tissue is embedded in a waxy block, and the plastic is peeled off. The technician places the block beneath a knobbed setscrew (right center). The assembly then cranks against a blade, shearing off thin sections of tissue.

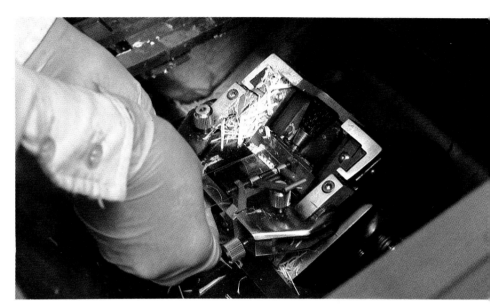

The technician next presses a microscope slide against one of the tissue cuttings. To be certain of selecting a representative sample, she may prepare two or three slides from the same frozen block and bring all of them to the pathologist.

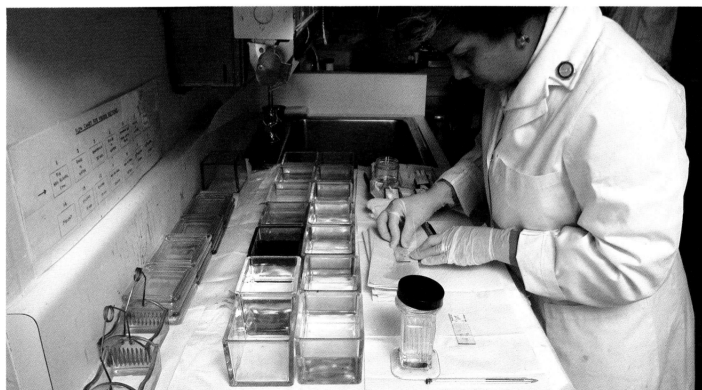

An adhesive identification-number tag is affixed to a slide after it has passed through the 14 chemical baths lined up in two rows on the counter. The deep-purple liquid at center left stains the nuclei of tissue cells for easier viewing; the orange bath at right rear highlights substances surrounding the nucleus. Other liquids remove fat, water and freezing solution from the tissue.

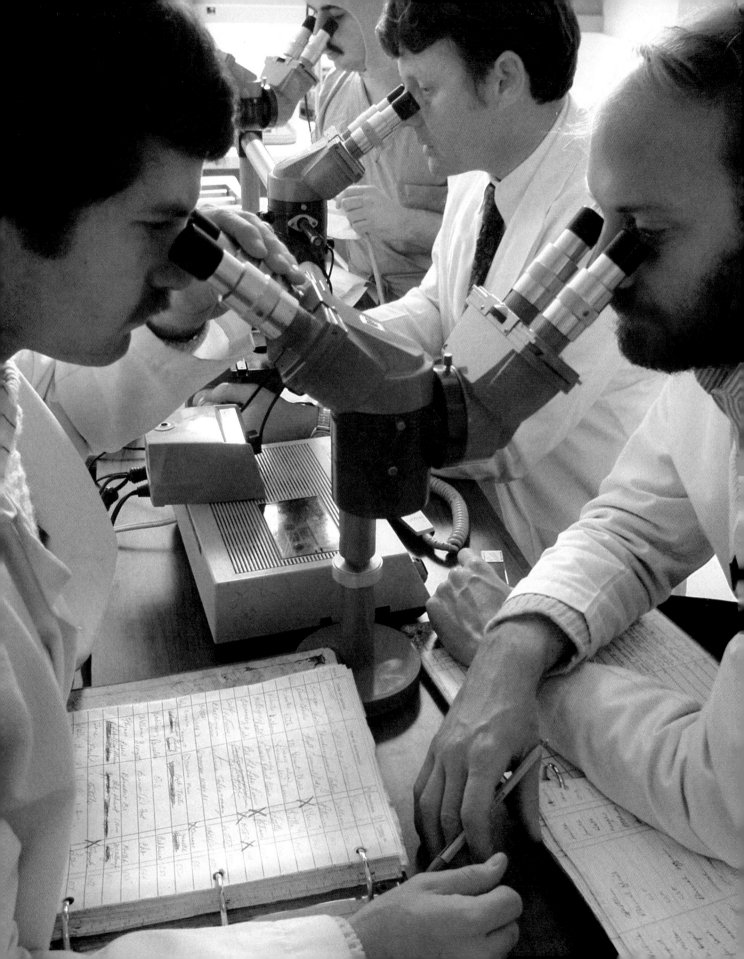

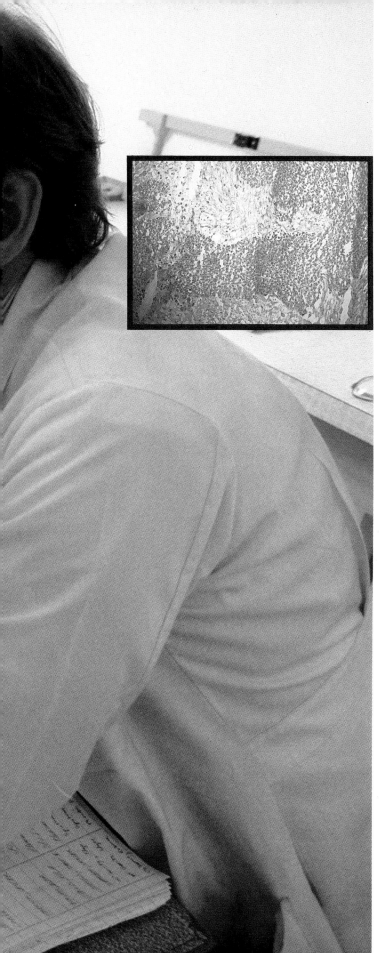

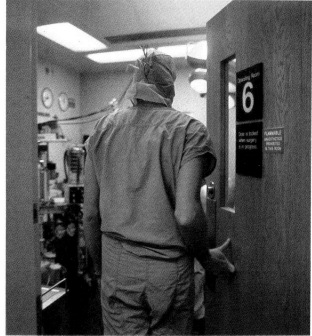

Seated before a microscope that is fitted with five sets of eyepieces, the pathologist (center) and his assistants discuss the appearance of cells in the frozen section, writing down their observations. Within about one minute, they reach a consensus, deciding from what they see whether the tumor is benign or malignant. In the case of the liver-tumor section reproduced in the inset, abnormally large, splotchy nuclei in the lower center section led to an inescapable conclusion: cancer.

A pathology assistant, wearing the sterile green of surgery, enters the operating room with the results of the biopsy. His report signals the waiting surgical team whether to go ahead and remove cancerous tissue—or simply to stitch up a small incision and send the patient out to the recovery room.

CHAPTER 4

Intimate profile of a wayward cell

Anatomy of the cell
Cancer that runs in families
A universal plan for all living things
The ticking time bomb of carcinogenesis
Viruses that cause cancer
The long search for a human cancer virus
How the body fights back

All cancers, whatever their cause, wherever in human tissue they erupt, are now known to begin at the most basic unit of life, at the level of a single cell. All of these malignancies, despite the great diversity of forms they take, despite the huge variations in their patterns of severity, begin as some infinitely subtle deviation in the growth cycle of just one cell among the 100 trillion or so making up the human body.

In seeking to find out what exquisite mechanisms, external or internal, can make a good cell go bad, researchers are now taking a closer look at the normal cell—what purpose it fulfills, how it is constructed, how its parts function, how its repair and replacement processes work. Knowledge of the normal cell is far from complete, but enough details have been discovered to raise the hope that the keys to cancer management lie there.

The cell is a marvel of microscopic organization. The smallest living unit capable of operating on its own in the body, it has three attributes that permit its relative independence. It has the ability to take in nutrients that have been broken down by the digestive system from ingested food; it has the skill to rearrange these simplified substances into the more complex compounds, chiefly proteins, necessary to energize and maintain it; and it has the capacity to produce new cells according to a pattern embedded in it. These crucial attributes are all manufacturing processes of unimaginable variety. In number and complexity, these processes present almost infinite opportunities for an error that can lead to the deviant cell growth of cancer.

The cell's capacities change with age, as might be expected. At conception, the very first cell that eventually will become a mature human being is formed in a unique way, through the union of male and female germ cells. Embedded in the male germ cell is the heredity pattern of the father; embedded in the female germ cell is the mother's pattern. Those two patterns intermingle during conception, producing a new pattern—unique to the forming baby—that is partly derived from each parent. Once this intermingling is accomplished at conception, the pattern that will govern cell reproduction in the future human being is normally fixed. Thus this first cell of a new life bears within it a plan for the production of all future cells. The first cell soon reproduces by dividing in two, passing the same characteristics along directly to each offspring cell; those two divide again, and so on and on.

At this early stage—and until shortly before birth—each dividing cell does not produce two exact copies of itself. Instead, as the cells multiply they change, specializing more and more to become brain cells, fingernail cells, liver cells and every other type of cell. When the body reaches maturity, most of its 100 trillion cells have differentiated in structure and capabilities to become working members of a functioning tissue. Some cells, however, never mature fully—the cells of bone marrow, for example, continue to differentiate into blood cells over a person's entire lifetime. Once cells have differentiated, they thereafter reproduce themselves exactly—so long as they remain healthy—each cell

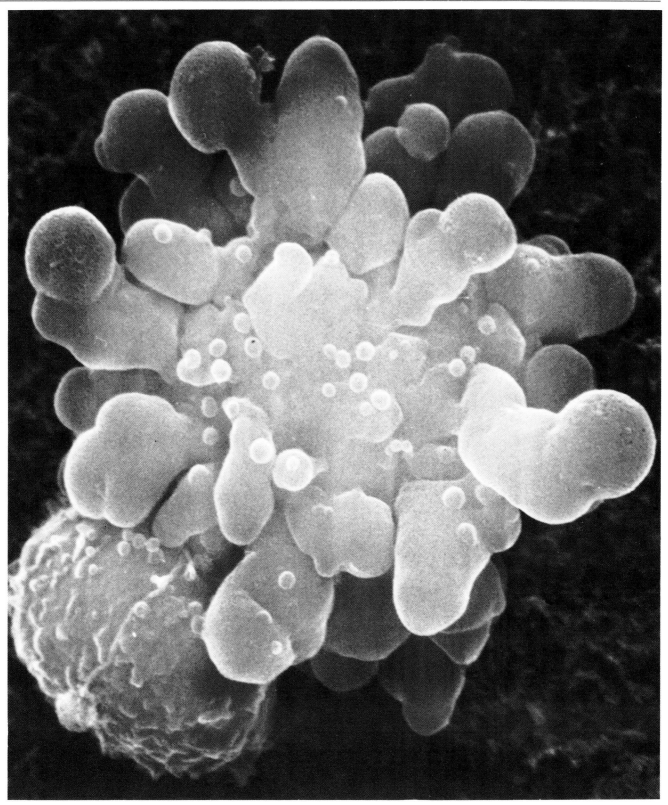

A tumor cell grown in mouse tissue disintegrates into harmless globules as it is attacked by a cell called a lymphocyte, visible at lower left in this scanning electron micrograph. Cancer-killing lymphocytes are among the many elements of the immune system, which defends against disease in animals and human beings.

dividing in two to make clones, identical copies of itself.

Some cells stop duplicating themselves after a while. The muscles that produce body movement acquire their maximum number of cells before birth; thereafter the muscles strengthen or weaken from changes in the size, not the number, of the cells. Brain cells multiply rapidly until birth and then begin to die off—thousands are lost each day; they are not replaced and mental capacity may eventually decrease. By contrast, some types of cells continue to reproduce so long as their owner lives—new cells of the skin, lung and mucous membranes, for example, steadily replace old ones that have worn out. Because cell reproduction is such a complex manufacturing process, so easily disrupted, the cells that are multiplying most rapidly are the ones that are most vulnerable to cancer.

Such differences in the reproductive capacities of cells account for differences in vulnerability to cancer from one part of the body to another. Brain cells, which practically stop multiplying at birth, almost never become cancerous—what is called cancer of the brain is really a malignancy that attacks not nerve cells but instead the supportive tissue, which does reproduce itself. For similar reasons, lung and skin cancers are very common because these cells must continually replace themselves.

Anatomy of the cell

Each type of cell has a characteristic form suited to its function. A skin cell is flat and flakelike; a liver cell is a small cube. Yet whatever the shape or function of a particular cell, it shares with every other cell a basic structure consisting of three major parts: an outer wrapper, called the cell membrane; the inner material, called the cytoplasm; and a core, called the nucleus.

The cell membrane is more than a container. It also acts as a gatekeeper, letting in certain nutrients and letting out waste materials and cell secretions. In addition, chemical sensors on the membrane surface act as controls: Malfunctioning sensors have been implicated in the spread of cancer. In a normal cell, these sensors ensure that the cell remains anchored in place and grows only to the boundaries of neigh-boring cells; when the population density reaches comfortable limits, a control known as contact inhibition causes cell division to cease. Together, the sensors are an assemblage of chemicals as unique to an individual as fingerprints, and they act as badges of membership; without these badges, a cell would be perceived as a strangeling by surrounding cells and attacked by a host of internal defense mechanisms.

The mouse that became a test tube

The hairless mouse pictured below is uniquely valuable to cancer research. But in 1962, when the first specimen turned up among experimental animals at a laboratory in Scotland, no one knew what to make of it. Then tests on its descendants led to a surprising discovery: Cells from certain human tumors, implanted in these mice, continued to grow. For the first time, scientists could study a human cancer cell in another animal, without risking a human life. One grateful scientist called the nude mouse "a test tube on four legs."

As it turned out, what makes the mouse a perfect host also makes it bald: It is born without a thymus gland, which would regulate its defenses against disease, and the same genetic accident that deprived it of the gland also destroyed its ability to grow hair. With a virtually limitless supply of the mice—one Boston facility raised 250,000 a year—researchers have been able to test an array of new drugs and radiation treatments, and doctors may soon be able to design treatment plans by trying alternative therapies on a series of nude mice.

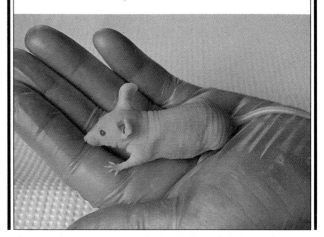

A tiny nude mouse rests on the hand of a technician at the National Institutes of Health in Rockville, Maryland. A sterile glove protects the mouse from infection; born without the normal defenses against disease, the animal would sicken and die of such ailments as mouse hepatitis in a normal environment.

Inside the cell membrane, the cytoplasm consists of water and a number of specialized structures. Like various departments of a factory, each of these structures makes its particular contribution along the production line toward the delivery of various chemical products. One structure functions chiefly as the cell's interdepartmental transport and communications system; another provides maintenance; still others supply the energy, packaging and warehousing for finished products. A structure known as a ribosome is charged with assembling the constantly arriving raw materials into the various protein substances the body needs for its physical upkeep and operation.

More than 30,000 different proteins are required. Whether they make up body parts, promote digestion, regulate growth or strengthen the immune system, all are produced out of just 20 different building blocks known as amino acids, which are relatively simple compounds present in food or manufactured from food by the cells.

Instructions for this intricate process are given by the nucleus, the third structural component of the cell. It, operating as the brains of the organization, is the site where most, if not all, cancer begins.

A round body poised somewhere near the center of the cell, the nucleus contains the huge, complex molecules of DNA—deoxyribonucleic acid—that control the physical traits in all forms of life. How the DNA is organized determines the form of an individual—whether it will be fly, frog or man, and if human, whether blond or dark.

Cancer that runs in families

All a human being's DNA is contained in 46 chromosomes, pairs of bow-shaped structures *(page 97),* one of each pair inherited from each parent. Within a chromosome, the DNA is divided into genes, each a portion of the DNA molecule containing a particular number and mix of molecular components, arranged in a particular sequence and located in a particular spot on the chromosome. It is the mix and sequence of these components that control the way a cell operates and multiplies. The control mechanism is passed along from parent cell to offspring cell—and thus from the parent human to the child—so that each healthy offspring cell functions in its prescribed manner. In this way DNA, by governing cell reproduction, governs the transmission of hereditary traits from parent to child.

Among those hereditary traits could be defective DNA that leads to cancer. There is some evidence that cancer runs in families, but because in most families all members are subjected to similar environmental influences, it is difficult to separate genetics from environment as a cause.

No such difficulty applies to animals, whose environments and heredity can be strictly controlled. And experiments in animal breeding demonstrate that a susceptibility to cancer can be inherited. Many varieties of laboratory mice, for example, have been crossbred to be peculiarly vulnerable to cancer, even to particular types of cancer.

Experiments with such mice led George J. Todaro and Robert J. Huebner of the National Cancer Institute to suggest that all adult vertebrates—every creature from lowly fish to humans—carry within their genetic material the potential code word for cancer. This gene, the researchers believe, was integrated into vertebrate DNA early in evolution as the result of some widespread viral infection, and it has remained there in a normally inactive state ever since. What triggers the activation of the inactive gene leading to the formation of a malignant tumor, they do not know, but if the cancer-coded gene is thought of as the sleeping carcinogenic initiator, it is easy to imagine that all sorts of environmental circumstances might awaken it.

Understanding how aberrant genes might lead to cancer requires a detailed knowledge of the DNA molecule itself. In 1944 Drs. Oswald T. Avery, Colin MacLeod and Maclyn McCarty of The Rockefeller Institute of New York identified DNA as the crucial compound in reproduction—and thus presumably in cancer.

DNA is a giant among molecules, an enormously long chemical chain constructed of somewhat smaller but still relatively large links. Each link is assembled from just three building blocks that are themselves parts of molecules. One is the type of compound classified as a sugar, similar to but simpler in structure than table sugar. The second is a phosphate group—the combination of a phosphorus atom with four atoms of oxygen. The third building block of any link can be any of four substances. Two of them, adenine and guanine, are relatively long molecules, constructed around two rings of atoms; they differ from each other in the number of oxygen atoms attached to one ring. The other two, cytosine and thymine, are smaller, one-ring structures; thymine contains one more oxygen atom than cytosine, and an extra group of carbon and hydrogen atoms. Thus each link in the DNA chain is made up of a sugar, a phosphate and either adenine, guanine, cytosine or thymine (usually identified by their initials: A, G, C and T).

Astonishingly, in this seemingly small compass of a few chemicals, all the information needed for the genetic variation in the living world is coded and compressed. How the code operates, however—and how garbling the code may initiate cancer—depends not on the ingredients in DNA but on their arrangement: the structure of the molecule.

A universal plan for all living things

Shortly after World War II many of the foremost scientists around the world plunged into an intense, often acerbic rivalry to figure out the structure of DNA. One reward for those who succeeded was certain to be a Nobel Prize. The investigators did not use the experimental mice, retorts and microscopes ordinarily involved in medical research, but one of the most abstruse techniques of science, X-ray diffraction. X-rays bounced off a crystal of DNA are reflected from its atoms in such a way that the rays interfere with one another. The interference creates a pattern of dots on a photographic plate, and complex mathematical analysis of such dot patterns could provide clues to the atomic arrangement creating the patterns. These clues could then be used to build toylike models out of wire and plastic balls—a physical structure that could be matched against the X-ray diffraction pattern of the real thing.

The race to discover the structure of DNA was won in 1953 by a brash young American biochemist doing postgraduate research at Cambridge University, James Watson, working with an only slightly older English physical chemist, Francis Crick. The two scientists shared a Nobel Prize in 1962.

Watson and Crick determined that DNA takes the form of a double helix, a paired spiral like a twisted rope ladder. The ropes of the DNA ladder are sugars and phosphates connected end to end. They are held together by ''rungs'' formed from joined pairs of the other components, A, G, C and T. The arrangement of these four in the rungs, Watson and Crick learned, is anything but random. Adenine, a longer molecule, is always paired with thymine, a shorter molecule, and the longer guanine is always found opposite and bonded to the shorter cytosine, so that the pairs are all the same width and the sides of the DNA ladder a uniform distance apart at every point. As for the spiral form, Watson and Crick concluded that it is a practical solution to a space problem. The DNA molecule, wound tighter than a coiled spring, jams an enormous amount of genetic material—some say the linear equivalent of a football field—into a nuclear space 1/10,000 the size of a pinhead.

With a few odd exceptions, each chromosome of each cell in the body contains a DNA molecule exactly like the one in the other chromosomes and cells. But only certain parts of any DNA molecule are active—the genes that contain particular groupings of DNA components. Each gene is unique in the sequence and numbers of the A-T and G-C pairings within it—as many as 4,000 in a single gene. Altogether there are some two million genes in every human cell; they are assembled in the offspring cell at the moment of sexual union and perpetuated, almost entirely without change, in every cell descendant thereafter.

Each cell's genes contain all the heritable information of the entire human organism—in effect, they are the complete instruction manual on how to make the proper cell type for the cornea, the lip, the spleen and every other part of the body. For each new cell to develop in its intended form, only the genes carrying the appropriate instructions must be read, and all the other genes must be ignored.

The average cell needs to manufacture (or ''express,'' as geneticists put it) less than 5 per cent of the proteins for which it has genes. The other 95 per cent or so of the genes remain ''repressed,'' so that they hold back all of their inappropriate

A fatal error inside a cell

Every cancer is the direct descendant of a single cell—one that was created unwholesomely different from normal cells. A normal cell, such as the one diagramed below, processes materials to carry out the work of the tissue or organ it is part of, to keep itself in repair and to reproduce by splitting in two. It performs these functions according to a detailed pattern passed down from earlier generations and stored in its genetic data bank, the complex DNA molecule.

Normally, when a mature cell divides, each new cell gets its own perfect copy of the parent DNA *(pages 98-99)*. But the DNA replication process occasionally misfires, producing a cell with a distorted genetic code. The descendants of that cell may not perform the functions they are supposed to but instead display unruly behavior, growing into malignant tumors that crowd out normal cells, obstruct their operations and siphon off their nutrients.

MEMBRANE SENSORS
Proteins on the cell's surface (symbolized by the hairlike projections in the drawing below, left) sense whether the cell should start or stop reproducing and whether it is in its proper location. In cancerous cells, the sensing functions may go awry.

PLASMA MEMBRANE
The cell's outer wrapping, a thin, flexible structure called the plasma membrane, regulates the entry of nutrients and the exit of wastes.

CYTOPLASM
Inside the membrane most of a cell is cytoplasm—a jelly-like pool in which float minute processing plants called organelles.

RIBOSOMES
Some organelles, called ribosomes, produce proteins. Ribosomes act on instructions; if the instructions are wrong—as in cancerous cells—the wrong kind or number of proteins will be produced, causing the cell to deviate from its intended form and functions.

NUCLEUS
The control center of a cell is its nucleus. Here a copy of the entire body's genetic code is kept, and from it come the instructions to the ribosomes.

CHROMOSOMES
The bow-shaped structures at left represent two of the 46 chromosomes that form in every normal human cell nucleus when the cell is preparing to divide. Chromosomes serve as a frame on which are fitted in precise order the chemical compounds that contain the genetic code.

DNA
Mounted on the chromosomes is deoxyribonucleic acid, the double-stranded spiral DNA *(above)* that is the substance of heredity in all life. The links between the spirals lie in distinctive sequences at particular sites on the chromosomes to spell out each organism's genetic code.

Order versus anarchy in reproduction

When a cell divides into two duplicates of itself, it must pass on two complete copies of DNA from its single copy. This is accomplished when the two strands of the original DNA break apart lengthwise and a new strand forms along each original. If duplication is to be accurate, the process requires great precision, for each segment of the completed DNA molecule is made up of four of the six available chemicals (symbolized at right): a phosphate and a sugar joined end to end for the strands, plus two of the four others for each link between strands.

The links must be assembled according to one strict rule: The long molecule called adenine (A) always pairs with the short thymine (T), and the long guanine (G) with the short cytosine (C). The pairs, themselves unvarying, appear along the DNA molecule in an almost infinite variety of sequences to spell out the individual's genetic code. When DNA carries the wrong genetic information, cancer may result.

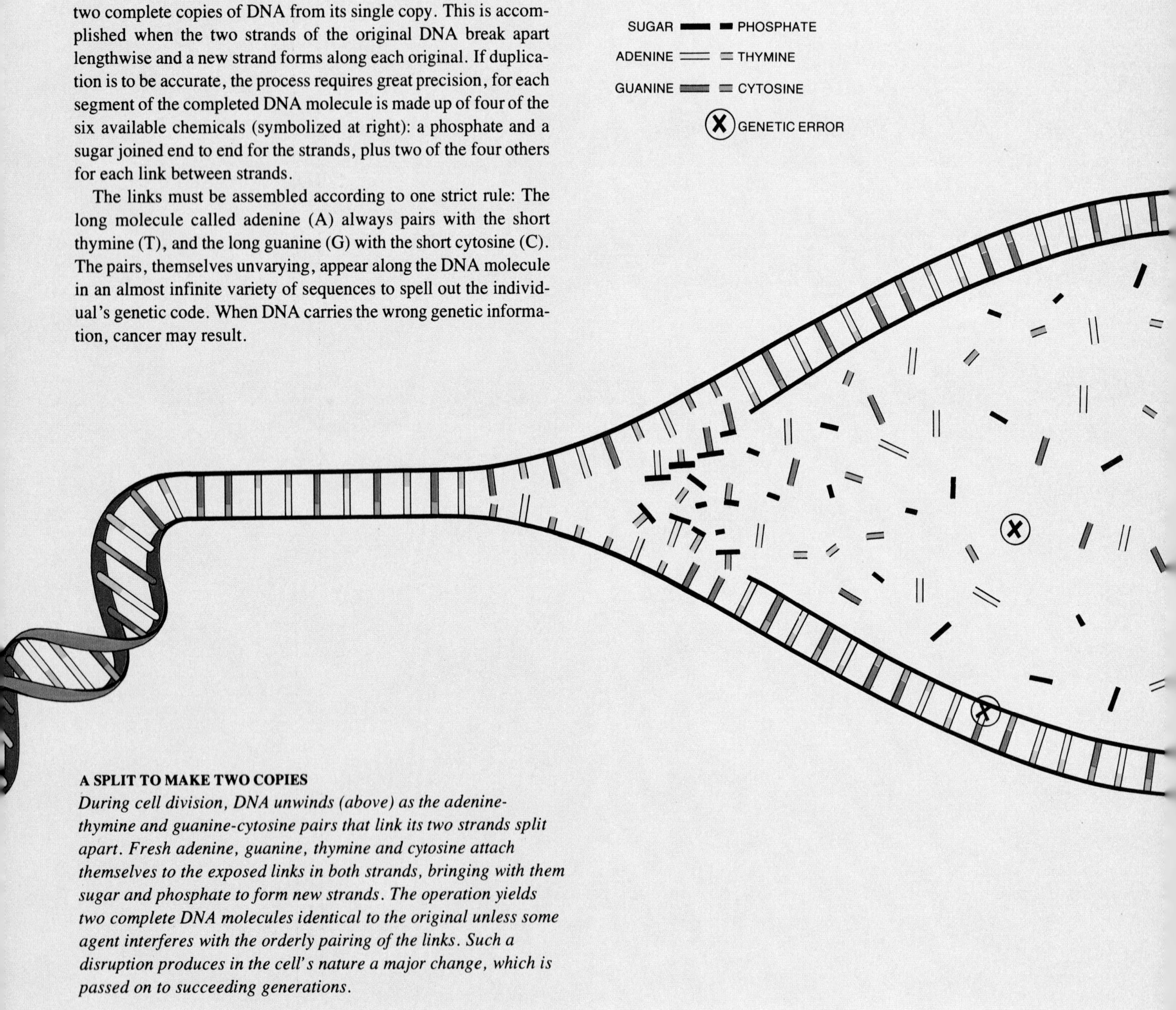

SUGAR ▬ ▬ PHOSPHATE
ADENINE ═ ═ THYMINE
GUANINE ▬ ═ CYTOSINE
Ⓧ GENETIC ERROR

A SPLIT TO MAKE TWO COPIES
During cell division, DNA unwinds (above) as the adenine-thymine and guanine-cytosine pairs that link its two strands split apart. Fresh adenine, guanine, thymine and cytosine attach themselves to the exposed links in both strands, bringing with them sugar and phosphate to form new strands. The operation yields two complete DNA molecules identical to the original unless some agent interferes with the orderly pairing of the links. Such a disruption produces in the cell's nature a major change, which is passed on to succeeding generations.

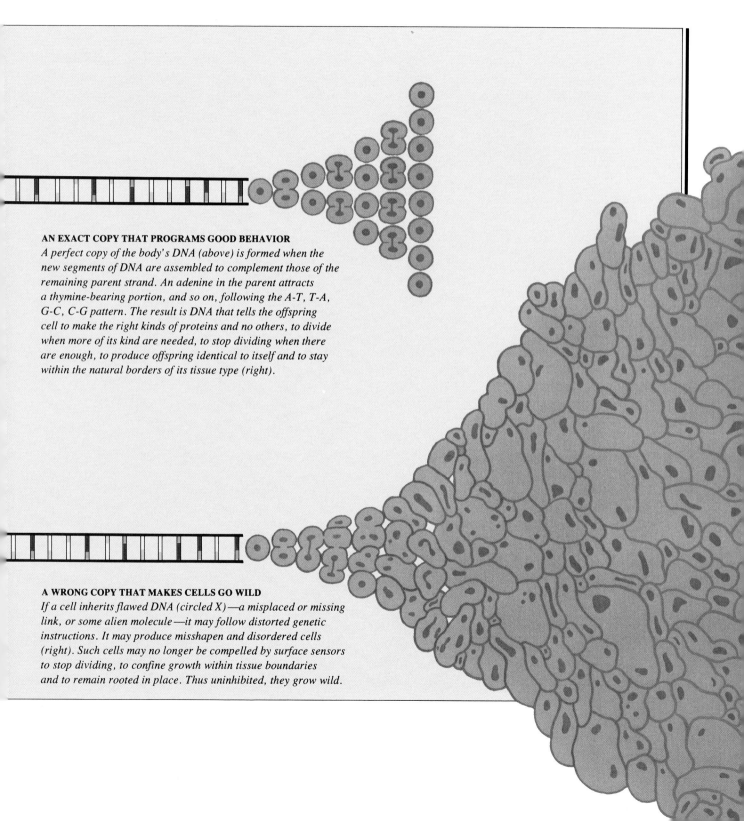

AN EXACT COPY THAT PROGRAMS GOOD BEHAVIOR

*A perfect copy of the body's DNA (above) is formed when the
new segments of DNA are assembled to complement those of the
remaining parent strand. An adenine in the parent attracts
a thymine-bearing portion, and so on, following the A-T, T-A,
G-C, C-G pattern. The result is DNA that tells the offspring
cell to make the right kinds of proteins and no others, to divide
when more of its kind are needed, to stop dividing when there
are enough, to produce offspring identical to itself and to stay
within the natural borders of its tissue type (right).*

A WRONG COPY THAT MAKES CELLS GO WILD

*If a cell inherits flawed DNA (circled X)—a misplaced or missing
link, or some alien molecule—it may follow distorted genetic
instructions. It may produce misshapen and disordered cells
(right). Such cells may no longer be compelled by surface sensors
to stop dividing, to confine growth within tissue boundaries
and to remain rooted in place. Thus uninhibited, they grow wild.*

instructions. The proteins for fingernails and toenails, for example, are coded in the DNA of every cell in the body but they are produced normally only by cells found at the ends of the fingers and toes.

The instructions expressed by the genes must be communicated to the cell's fabrication department—the ribosomes—if they are to manufacture new proteins of the proper type. The messenger that carries the instructions is another complex chemical compound, in this case ribonucleic acid. RNA, as it is called, is quite similar chemically to DNA, except that its sugar component has one less oxygen molecule. From this difference comes RNA's structural difference—it typically takes the form of a single rather than a double spiral. RNA performs a variety of jobs, but its most significant one in terms of the cancer connection is thought to be its messenger function.

Building new life

In a process still only partially understood, messenger RNA is produced in the nucleus. A short stretch of the DNA double spiral flattens and spreads apart, exposing a section of rungs that constitutes a gene. Free molecules in the nucleus attach to the exposed DNA, forming a portion of RNA—a single strand that is a mirror image of the bit of DNA that made it. When the messenger RNA is completed, it breaks away from its DNA template and leaves the nucleus to enter the cytoplasm. It then attaches itself to a ribosome. There, with the help of other forms of RNA, it initiates manufacture of the specific protein for which it is patterned.

This process of sending instructions via RNA to the ribosome protein factories governs the manufacture of materials the cell needs and also of materials to produce a new cell. A new cell needs something more—a complete DNA molecule properly coded so that the offspring can, in its turn, reproduce as intended.

Transmission of the organism's entire genetic code to the next generation of cells, part of the process of cell division, is accomplished in somewhat similar fashion to that used for generating messenger RNA. When a cell is preparing to divide, the double helix of DNA separates into two single flat strands, and the A-T and G-C pairs split. Each section then acts as a template, against which molecules line up. These form a new complementary strand in the image of the one that was lost—a section of the code reading, for example, A-T-G-C-C-T automatically providing the pattern for a newly created sequence of T-A-C-G-G-A, and so on.

The production of this new mirror-image DNA strand may take as long as 10 hours, and minor errors occasionally occur. A portion may be copied more than once, or bits of the code may be transcribed in some inverted order; but the cell contains substances that make small corrections along the way. When the copying process is complete, the cell has enough genetic material for two new daughter cells. The dividing cell then concludes its life cycle by splitting into two fully independent cell units, each ready to repeat the exact cell cycle all over again, each a perfect clone of the now-nonexistent parent cell.

Perfect, that is, unless some rare event, sufficient to overtax the nucleus's normal repair mechanisms, comes along. One of the possible consequences of such an event is heritable changes in cell chemistry.

Such changes can be of several types. Genes may become permanently altered because one or more of the DNA components are lost, rearranged or replaced with a substitute. The cause of such a mutation may be a chance error or an external agent causing damage to the DNA. The effect can range from a simple change in a single link in the chain, barely detectable by even the most advanced techniques of biomedical observation, to a gross change, called a frame shift, in which the addition or subtraction of one or more links on one strand of the DNA molecule causes a one-sided bulge in the double spiral. This alteration can have a ripple effect on scores, perhaps hundreds, of neighboring genes as the links between the two strands become mismatched all the way down the line and the A's, T's, G's and C's on one strand are forced to form new bonds with complements that are many notches below or above their proper site. Such a frame shift either kills the cell or produces cancer.

A second kind of change occurs when alien genetic material—genes from some other living creature—infiltrates the

The immortal cells of Henrietta Lacks

Henrietta Lacks *(right)*, a Baltimore wife and mother, died of cervical cancer in 1951. To all appearances, her death was but one more cancer tragedy. But there was something different about Henrietta Lacks's cancer. Cells from her tumor, preserved in a laboratory dish at The Johns Hopkins University Hospital, survived and reproduced themselves. For the first time in scientific history human cancer cells had prospered outside a living body.

The news quickly spread. Over the next few years HeLa cells—named for their donor—were sent to laboratories around the world. Quick to reproduce and easy to work with, they were used in almost every kind of cell research, including the development of the Salk polio vaccine. Henrietta Lacks had gained a kind of immortality—but it proved a bane as well as a blessing.

In 1966 Dr. Stanley Gartner of the University of Washington made a troubling discovery. Experimental cultures of human cells, believed to be from different tissues and individuals, were HeLa cells, identifiable by certain cellular components. During the early years of work, HeLa cells had gotten into other tissue cultures, multiplied furiously and replaced the original cells. In the years following this discovery, a team of researchers led by Dr. Walter Nelson-Rees at the University of California identified more than 100 such contaminated cell cultures. Samples supposed to be kidney, bladder, breast and prostate cells, for example, were found to be mainly HeLa cervix cells—after the results of research on the tissues had been widely accepted.

Some cancer research performed during the late 1950s and early 1960s had to be reevaluated; months of work, much money—and some hard-earned reputations—were lost. One theory—the spontaneous transformation into cancer of human cells growing normally in a culture—was shot down. The cultures in which spontaneous transformation occurred apparently had been not normal at all, but contaminated with HeLa cells; today, the transformation phenomenon is considered very rare, if it occurs at all.

Fortunately, most of the research on the HeLa-contaminated cultures was in basic biology and is not in doubt. The nature of the cells—whether kidney or cervix—had little or nothing to do with the results. And since the mid-1960s, laboratory procedures have been refined to prevent contamination, so that the great discoveries of succeeding years are not under suspicion. Henrietta Lacks's living and apparently immortal legacy, now under control, serves again as an invaluable laboratory tool.

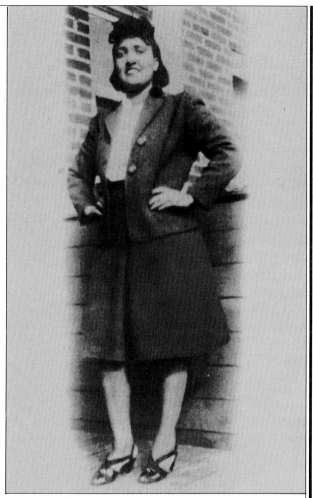

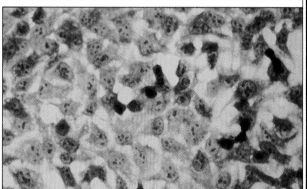

Henrietta Lacks, in her late twenties in the picture at top, died at the age of 31, from a cervical cancer characterized by what are now known as HeLa cells (above). The cells, marked by the dense growth and oversized or multiple nuclei common in cancer tissue, have a unique ability to flourish in laboratory cultures.

cell's normal DNA. The agent for this sort of mutation is thought to be a virus.

Still another mechanism of mutation is caused not by a change in the number or position of genes but in the way the correct genes, particularly those cast in a repressor role, behave. In this kind of mutation, some of the genes that have for generations remained repressed may suddenly begin to be expressed, while others, essential to normal function, somehow are suddenly turned off. The telltale sign of such a mutation is that the cell loses its specialized nature, its unique tissue characteristics, and regresses toward some embryonic state. Some degree of "dedifferentiation," as cell biologists call this trend, is a common characteristic of many kinds of cancer cells.

However, even these large-scale disruptions of DNA are generally harmless—they cause a spot or lump that, if detectable at all, is innocuous. The differences between such benign tumors and malignant ones are generally obvious, although as any cancer specialist knows, the lines of distinction are not nearly as finite in practice as might be wished. Some benign tumors occasionally evolve into a malignant state over time, and some tumors exhibiting intermediate features of malignancy fail to develop further. And in very rare instances, distinctly cancerous cells revert to a normal state.

Benign or cancerous, a tumor cell behaves quite differently from a normal cell in a number of critical ways. Principally, it becomes autonomous, meaning that it is no longer subject to the usual control mechanisms that make a normal cell a cooperative, social being within a community of tissue cells. The autonomy, once established, becomes a heritable trait, passed on to each new generation of cells. Benign tumors are relatively minor offenders of the social order. Most remain in place and do not migrate. Their structural deviation is slight, so that they continue to be recognizable as descendants of the normal cell from which they sprang. They usually grow slowly and can be left alone.

Malignant-tumor cells are, by contrast, given to behavior that ranges from the antisocial to the anarchic. In size and structure these rogue cells may be so aberrant that they no longer resemble their original tissue type. Dedifferentiating,

they lose particular qualities that were essential to their functioning. The nucleus becomes irregular, large and active—often at the expense of an undersized cytoplasm. They persist in reproducing themselves without regard to the usual constraints of cell population density, sometimes invading neighboring tissue. More dangerous still, they have a tendency to override anchorage dependence, the constraints that keep most cells attached in one location. Breaking loose from their original site, they travel through the bloodstream or lymph system to sometimes distant locations, where they may start up new colonies of secondary cancer, a spread called metastasis.

The cell disruptions of cancer are concentrated largely in one particular type of cell—the epithelial cells, which cover the skin and other tissues, make up glandular organs such as the breast, and line the lungs and gastrointestinal tract. These disruptions generate the type of cancer known as carcinomas, which account for more than 85 per cent of all cancers. Unlike the other main types—sarcomas of the connective and supportive tissue, leukemias of the blood, and lymphomas of the lymph system—carcinomas increase in incidence with age. The reason may be related to the fact that epithelial cells are by nature the ones most frequently and persistently exposed to the external chemical, physical and viral agents that are labeled carcinogens.

An alarming list of carcinogens has been compiled over the centuries since Dr. Percivall Pott noted a relationship between scrotal cancer among English chimney sweeps and their exposure to the tars in chimney soot. The list grows longer almost every day. It includes not only man-made substances such as the soot from fires and the tongue-twisting chemicals of modern plastics, but also natural agents such as sunlight and the ingredients in traditional, unadulterated foods *(Chapter 2)*.

The ticking time bomb of carcinogenesis

Why carcinogens, such as coal tars and vinyl chloride, cause cancer but other substances do not is still something of a mystery. But how they accomplish their deadly sabotage of a cell's DNA is becoming understood. Many authorities believe that this induction of cancer, this carcinogenesis, is often a two-stage process. In the first stage, initiation, a potentially carcinogenic substance makes its way into the body—eaten in food, breathed with air or absorbed through the skin. At this point the carcinogen is carried, either unchanged or in some modified form, to a cell. The invader's molecules add, subtract or substitute something in the cell's DNA, or repress or activate certain genes, altering the messages sent from the nucleus to the ribosome protein factories.

While a single exposure to some carcinogens can initiate unusually rapid tumor formation, more often the affected cell and its abnormal progeny reproduce at more or less the same rate as the normal cells around them. They cause little if any disruption of the tissue and thus produce no changes that would be noticed. It takes a promoter to jar the altered cells into dangerously rapid and uncontrolled reproduction; without this promotion it is theoretically possible for potential cancer cells to remain no more explosive than a dynamite charge without a fuse.

The promoter is often some physical irritation that stimulates rapid cell replacement in the region where the abnormal cells reside. For example, certain chemicals that are not in themselves carcinogens can kill some cells; this destruction is almost always followed by a compensatory effort by surrounding cells to reproduce themselves and replace those that are lost. Promotion of cancer can come at any time—within weeks after carcinogenic initiation or many years later—but once it happens the abnormal cells begin to divide in a profligate manner.

A dramatic illustration of the interrelationship of initiation and promotion was provided by an experiment reported in 1947 by Drs. Philippe Shubik and Isaac Berenblum at Oxford University, in England. They applied a minute dose of dimethylbenzanthracene, or DMBA, one of the known carcinogenic components of tar, to the skin of a group of mice. They then separated the mice into two study groups, immediately daubing the skin of one group with a blistering agent known as croton oil (the promoter), and painting the other group with the same oil after a lapse of 16 weeks. Almost every mouse in both groups developed a tumor. In still other

groups of mice, no tumors arose when either the DMBA initiator or the croton-oil promoter was administered alone, nor did any develop if the promoter preceded the initiator in order of treatment. Evidence of this sort suggests that the sequence of cell change (initiation) followed by irritation and cell death (promotion) followed by rapid cell replacement makes up a rigidly orchestrated process that must always be played out in the same order, however variable the tempo, if cancer is to occur.

Why rapid cell replacement should promote tumor formation rather than simple tissue repair is still a matter of some speculation. One possible explanation is based on conventional laws of inheritance governing recessive genes, which generally remain inactive unless they are paired. Cancer-inducing genes are ordinarily recessive, but they could become active, or dominant, and begin producing abnormal quantities of proteins if, during cell division, both halves of the normally dividing chromosomes mistakenly end up in the same nucleus. When this happens, a pair of recessive genes is made dominant.

Such accidental gene pairings must be rare, but they might occur more frequently if cell replacement is accelerated. If the overall theory of initiation-promotion in most cancers turns out to be accurate, it may help explain the alarming increase in cancer during the past century. The theory implies that a great many natural carcinogens have existed in the environment throughout human history but have remained inactive, like bombs that have never exploded. Today, however, is a time of intense chemical innovation—some 1,000 new compounds are invented every year in the United States alone. It is easy to imagine that a few of these compounds, however innocent in their own right, can have a promotional effect on some potentially cancerous cell that might otherwise remain dormant.

Viruses that cause cancer

The processes of initiation and promotion also seem to be at work when a virus rather than a chemical is to blame for cancer. Viruses have long been known to induce animal cancers, but their involvement in human forms of the disease was not established until 1964, with the identification of one virus that apparently causes an unusual jaw cancer in African children, Burkitt's lymphoma *(pages 104-105)*.

The existence of viruses as agents of disease was first hinted at in 1892 by Dimitri Ivanovski, a Russian bacteriologist who was studying tobacco mosaic disease in tobacco plants. General belief at the time held that bacteria, still something of a novelty themselves, would eventually prove to be responsible for mosaic disease and for every other infection as well. But Ivanovski was unable to isolate any blameworthy bacteria under his microscope. He then tried an experiment with the sap drawn from a diseased plant. He passed the fluid through the newly developed porcelain filters that Louis Pasteur and others had shown would stop the smallest known bacteria, and then introduced the filtrate into healthy plants. To Ivanovski's surprise, the healthy plants became infected, apparently by some unknown agent of tobacco mosaic disease so small that it had gone through a bacteria-proof filter.

Over the next several decades other scientists went on to link a range of mysterious diseases in both plants and animals to this new class of filterable organisms. By the time these organisms, dubbed viruses, were made visible by the invention of the electron microscope in 1933, influenza, herpes infections, poliomyelitis and a legion of other human infections had been added to the list of virus-induced diseases—and by 1964, so was cancer.

A virus is an odd creature, existing somewhere in the twilight zone between living creatures and lifeless materials. Perhaps hundreds of times smaller than most bacteria, a thousand times smaller than the cell it infects, the virus looks more like an inert crystal than anything in the biological world. It also lacks such seemingly essential attributes as the ability to propel itself, to eat and digest nutrients, and to reproduce on its own.

In its structure, the virus is like a miniature cell nucleus stripped of its surrounding cytoplasm. Except for a protective coat of protein molecules, it is nothing but a tiny amount of DNA or RNA coded for as few as three to as many as hundreds of genes. But with these few genes, it operates as a

Trophy of a doctor's safari: the long-sought cancer virus

Though viruses have been known since 1908 to cause cancer in animals, it remained for an Irish surgeon, Denis Burkitt, a Colonial Service officer in Uganda in the 1950s, to connect human cancer and a virus. The culprit turned out to be common herpes virus, which in one form brings on nothing worse than cold sores.

Burkitt had been seeing a jaw cancer in Ugandan children for years. But he did not know what to make of a five-year-old boy with swellings on both sides of both jaws. "I didn't think it was a tumor," the surgeon recalled. "Nobody is likely to have four tumors at once." Soon he saw more similar swellings, and eventually they were indeed identified as cancer tumors, an unusual form of a malignancy of the lymph nodes *(pages 106-107)* now known as Burkitt's lymphoma.

Burkitt was intrigued by several characteristics of the disease. It occurred in clusters and seemed confined to parts of Africa—suggesting an infection related to environment. To find just where

the lymphoma was prevalent, he sent picture leaflets to missions and hospitals, asking if the condition had been seen. And in 1961, he set out on a 10-week, 10,000-mile safari, visiting 57 hospitals in 12 countries to locate lymphoma cases. His trip confirmed replies to his mail surveys, pinpointing a tumor swath across equatorial Africa and down the east coast—a hot, humid region plagued by mosquitoes that spread malaria and viruses.

Burkitt's findings stirred laboratory researchers around the world to look for a virus in samples of the lymphoma. It was found in 1964 by Dr. M. A. Epstein, Yvonne Barr and B. G. Achong of Middlesex Hospital in London: a type of herpes now named Epstein-Barr virus. It is no more common in Africa than elsewhere, but it causes Burkitt's lymphoma principally there because its cancerous effect must be triggered by an infection such as mosquito-borne malaria—which is far more common in Africa than in most other parts of the world.

perfect parasite when it comes in contact with a suitable host cell. Delivered there after entering the body by various means—skin contact, ingestion with food, respiration, insect bite—the virus penetrates a cell membrane and takes command of cell operations. It compels cellular management and labor to cease their normal activities and attend to its coded instructions. The instructions are to make more viruses—or to produce cancerous cells.

The long search for a human cancer virus

Even before viruses had a name, their involvement in animal cancers was recognized. In 1911 Peyton Rous of The Rockefeller Institute for Medical Research gathered bacteria-free fluids from chicken tumors and transmitted them to several healthy chickens; the chickens soon developed tumors of their own. Since then, virus-caused cancers have been identified in many kinds of birds and mammals.

Many human cancers also suggest a virus origin, mainly because cases occur in concentrated geographical pockets, as though caused by the spread of infection. One such cluster aroused concern in 1978 with the outbreak of Hodgkin's disease and leukemia in Rutherford, New Jersey, a suburb of New York City. In that year 19 cases of Hodgkin's disease and 13 cases of leukemia were diagnosed there, more than would normally be expected in a town with Rutherford's 21,000 population. Yet despite careful investigation, no connection to a virus could be found. Nor have similar small-scale epidemics of common cancers been linked to infectious agents of any kind.

However, it was the clustering of a very rare jaw cancer, Burkitt's lymphoma, among children of one area of Africa that led to its virus cause, the special form of the common herpes organism called Epstein-Barr virus. This virus occurs everywhere and is believed to infect almost everyone in the world at some time or another. Blood tests of American students revealed that between 35 and 80 per cent of them had been attacked by the virus before they entered college—and 10 to 15 per cent of those who had not were infected every year thereafter.

Most of these invasions by Epstein-Barr virus cause no

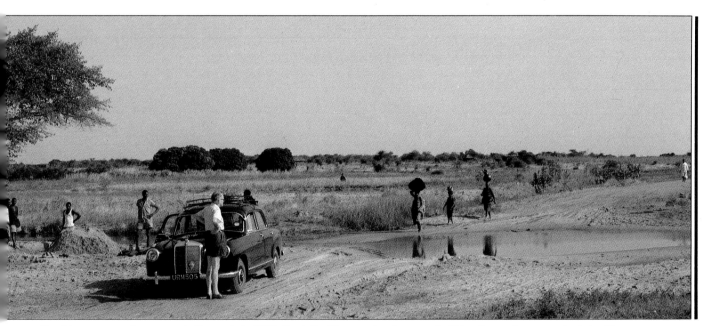

Tracking a strange jaw cancer in Tanzania in 1964, Denis Burkitt stops to ask passersby if they know of any cases in their villages.

A drainage system that helps and harms

Within the circulatory system, along with the arteries, veins and capillaries that carry blood out to tissues and back to the heart, is a subsidiary set of vessels and organs known as the lymph system. It performs a number of widely varying jobs, several of them crucial in the development of a cancer. Mainly, the lymph system is a drainage network that picks up materials released by body tissues and transports them to the bloodstream. In that role it may spread cancer. But it also is a mainstay of the body's defense system, isolating and neutralizing disease agents—including cancer.

As a transport network, the lymph system absorbs fluid surrounding tissue cells and carries it through ever larger vessels to each side of the neck, where connections to veins dump the fluid into the bloodstream. This lymph fluid, which is 95 per cent water and originates in the blood, contains wastes from healthy cells and harmful substances such as cancer cells to be disposed of. Other components of lymph are essential materials that must be distributed to meet body needs. Among them are disease-combating white blood cells produced by bone marrow, spleen, thymus and tonsils.

In addition, the lymph system produces white cells of its own in tiny organs called nodes. The nodes also serve as filters, trapping bacteria, virus-infected cells and plain dirt for elimination by the white blood cells there; the "swollen glands" that can accompany influenza are lymph nodes enlarged as they filter out virus-infected cells. The same filtering process stops or slows the spread of cancer cells.

A COLLECTING NETWORK
Lymph vessels (green) return lymph— blood fluid that has delivered its nourishment and now contains cell products—to the bloodstream both through protective nodes (dots) and through the thoracic and right lymphatic ducts.

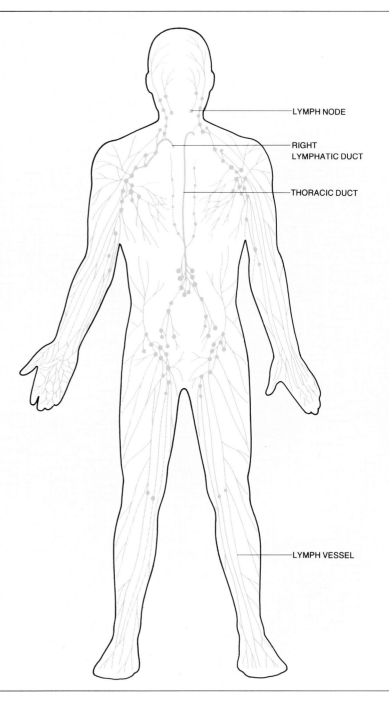

LYMPH NODE

RIGHT LYMPHATIC DUCT

THORACIC DUCT

LYMPH VESSEL

TWO INTERLOCKING SYSTEMS

The vessels (green) returning lymph to the blood interlace with blood vessels (red and blue) throughout the body but connect directly only to veins near the neck. Fluid enters the lymph system from tissue space around lymph capillaries (inset, bottom).

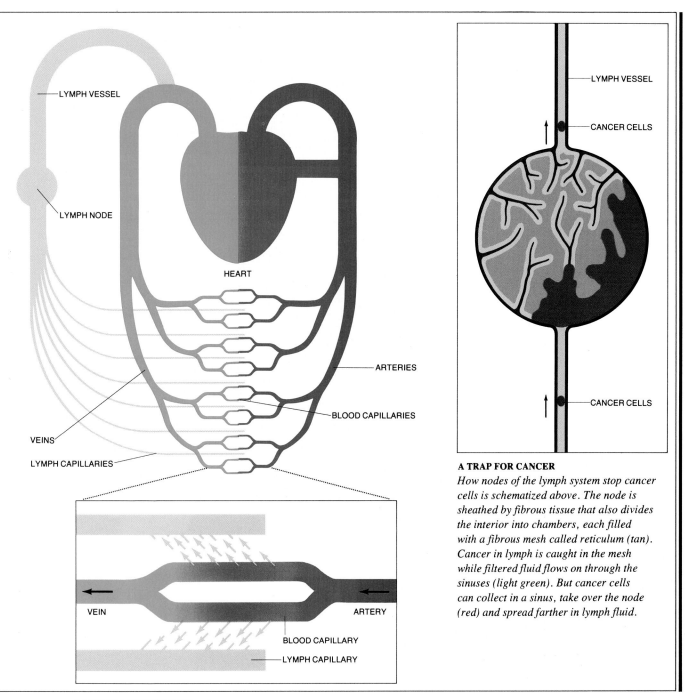

A TRAP FOR CANCER

How nodes of the lymph system stop cancer cells is schematized above. The node is sheathed by fibrous tissue that also divides the interior into chambers, each filled with a fibrous mesh called reticulum (tan). Cancer in lymph is caught in the mesh while filtered fluid flows on through the sinuses (light green). But cancer cells can collect in a sinus, take over the node (red) and spread farther in lymph fluid.

A MEDIUM OF EXCHANGE

Through an artery and blood capillaries, blood reaches a tissue bed, where capillaries release fluid (arrows) to feed cells and absorb cell products. Then part of the fluid passes into lymph capillaries, which pick up large molecules such as proteins, leaving simpler ones to be removed mainly by vein capillaries.

harm; when they do, the result in temperate climates is generally mononucleosis, the debilitating but nonfatal illness of young adults—called the kissing disease because Epstein-Barr virus is spread by mouth-to-mouth contact. The virus almost never leads to jaw cancer except in Africa, but it has also been implicated in a rare nose cancer occurring in scattered areas around the globe—southern China, Alaska, Tunisia and East Africa.

Thus Epstein-Barr virus seems to be an initiator—an infection that does not produce cancer unless stimulated by a promoter. The promoter apparently is another infection, not necessarily viral. In the lymphoma-stricken regions of Africa, it is presumably malaria, which is caused by a parasite spread by mosquitoes. Other infections must also be promoters, for even Burkitt's lymphoma occasionally appears in areas where malaria is unknown.

How the body fights back

The rarity of the jaw and nose cancers, despite the prevalence of Epstein-Barr virus, is testimony to the effectiveness of the body's natural defenses against disease, the immune system. It automatically goes into action to fight off any disturbance, mobilizing a defensive array of white blood cells, chemicals and filters. Some of these elements recognize a foreign substance—viruses, bacteria and all kinds of malignant cells as well as anything else that does not belong in the body. Other parts of the immune system then spread the alarm, trap the invader and kill it.

Leukemia cells, for example, have been found to carry on their surfaces chemical markers called antigens—substances that the body perceives as not part of the self, or foreign. (Every cell also carries certain markers that establish its right to be in the particular tissue of a particular body.) The most common sorts of antigens are the protein and carbohydrate markers that are worn like scarlet letters on viruses and bacteria, but a great variety of alien chemical compounds also mimic the antigen markers.

The antigens stimulate the body to produce antibodies—substances that block the spread of the disease agent. Each antibody is specific, working against only one kind of agent;

the body is signaled to make that particular antibody by the antigen marker on the invader.

Antigens also stimulate the thymus gland and the lymph system *(pages 106-107)* to release a special variety of white blood cells called T cells. They destroy foreign cells, including cancers, on contact.

A third element in the immune system's response to cancer—and one that seems to be independent of antibodies and T cells—is the natural killer cell, presumably a kind of white blood cell. It is believed to be present normally in the lymph system, but its effectiveness is enhanced by interferon, a substance that serves as an all-purpose defense agent. The attack of a virus, for example, makes a cell release a few molecules of interferon, but those few molecules are enough to arouse effective defense of the entire body. In test-tube experiments, 1/30,000,000,000,000 ounce of interferon will knock out half a million virus-infected cells.

Altogether the various parts of the immune system keep up a constant surveillance of the body. Stopping literally millions of random assaults that every human being sustains annually, letting very few diseases take hold, the system can be said to function extremely well most of the time. Many budding tumors, oncologists believe, are intercepted and destroyed by the immune system. But the system, though nearly perfect, is not totally perfect. Something must go wrong to

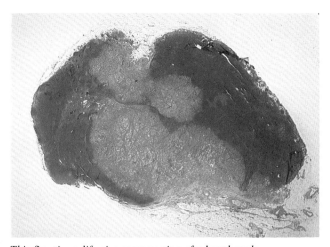

This five-times-life-size cross section of a lymph node— which filters disease agents, including cancerous cells, from body fluids—reveals it to be almost completely filled with malignant cells (light fibrous area). A node clogged by cancer can filter no more, causing cancer cells to overflow to another node nearby.

permit the rare cancer cell to survive and proliferate in the midst of so many bodyguards.

Immune systems, it is now apparent, vary considerably in effectiveness from one individual to the next. To some extent this difference is a matter of inheritance, which determines the quality of the immunological equipment that each person is born with, just as it determines fingerprints, blood type and facial characteristics. To some extent it is a matter of age. The older an individual is, the greater the likelihood that his immune system will develop deficiencies and weaknesses—and this at a time when his cells are experiencing the cumulative effects of years of exposure to carcinogens together with ever-increasing numbers of copying errors in the production of new cellular DNA.

In some cases, the immune system may itself be so taxed by some other illness as to have no margin left over for dealing with a rogue cancer cell.

Conversely, anything that would strengthen the immune system seems likely to help against cancer. There is evidence that protection against cancer can be stimulated this way, and some of the research was done long before the complexities of immunity were even partly understood.

Before the turn of the century, Dr. William Bradford Coley, a somewhat eccentric New York surgeon, devised a last-ditch treatment for patients suffering from inoperable cancers. Observing that a cancer victim in his care had experienced a marked shrinkage of a neck tumor after contracting a facial skin infection, he was inspired to see what might happen if he administered a mixture of bacterial toxins to his most hopeless patients. Many found themselves brought close to a premature death, with chills, fever and muscle aches, but most did eventually recover from the "cure"—and their tumors were considerably reduced in size and seriousness. In one remarkable case a 16-year-old boy with what was diagnosed as a fatal tumor actually watched his cancer disappear completely.

The effects of "Coley's toxins" were generally dismissed as coincidences at best and as quackery at worst. Little was heard of the technique for nearly three quarters of a century. Then, in 1972, cancer statisticians at the Albany Medical Center in New York noted that, contrary to expectations, lung cancer patients who had suffered postoperative lung infections ultimately showed a higher-than-average rate of recovery from cancer than those with no surgical infection. Similar relationships were noted in a large sample of Canadian youngsters: Those given a live tuberculosis vaccine known as BCG as part of a program of childhood immunization subsequently experienced a far lower rate of leukemia occurrence than those who had not been vaccinated.

Research in the years since has led immunologists to believe that these results indicate an immune response in which interferon stimulates the killer type of white blood cells. Although interferon was initially recognized, in 1957, to be a protection against virus infections, soon it was found to work against cancer—at least in animals—whether the cancer was caused by a virus, a chemical or radiation. When interferon was injected into cancer-stricken animals, it attacked tumor cells, inhibiting their growth, and it also stimulated other anticancer activities of the natural immune system.

Attempts to produce interferon for experimental treatments at first met almost insuperable difficulties. Dr. Kari Cantell of Helsinki worked out a way to separate one type of human interferon from blood donated at the Finnish Red Cross Blood Transfusion Center; in 1978 he processed 11,250 gallons of human blood to obtain 1,200 gallons of crude interferon—but those 1,200 gallons contained only 1/300 ounce of the pure chemical. By 1980, however, biochemists had achieved a coup of genetic engineering that promised unlimited supplies; they manipulated DNA molecules of certain bacteria so that cultures of bacteria cells would manufacture human interferon in vats.

Whatever uses will be found for interferon and other stimulants of the immune system, they will doubtless come, as will every other tool of cancer control and therapy, out of a growing accumulation of experiments in the behavior of cells, both normal and cancerous. Theories, some seemingly conservative, some wildly imaginative, still outnumber facts in many areas. Only when a way has been found to destroy the last cancer cell in the last cancer victim can it truly be said that the science of cancer care is complete. ✳

Saving lives with killer rays

In a floor plan of the Radiation Therapy Division at The Johns Hopkins Oncology Center in Baltimore, Maryland, the rooms where cancer patients are treated seem planned for a fortress. The walls are six feet of solid concrete with eight inches of steel embedded in them. Ceilings are five and a half feet of concrete and contain three inches of steel. Doors, thinner than the walls so that they are light enough to be opened and closed, are behind overlapping walls, as they were in medieval strongholds. This massive protection is needed to thwart a danger that can never be seen and seldom be felt—the radiation, generally X-rays, that kills cancer cells but also can harm healthy tissue. Some beams are so potent that direct exposure for two to three minutes can be fatal.

Such rooms are not unique to Johns Hopkins. They are necessary in any hospital to prevent the rays that both heal and harm from escaping treatment areas and endangering people nearby. And inside the heavily shielded enclosures, special steps must be taken to protect the very patients who are the intended targets of the beams. Unavoidably, some healthy tissue is damaged by radiation as it enters the body on the way to the tumor and again as the rays make their exit. To minimize this danger, a beam can be narrowed for small tumors or widened for extensive ones; shields custom-made for each patient safeguard areas next to the tumor.

Initially, each course of treatment is planned on simulators, which emit low-powered X-rays and harmless light beams *(right)*. Computers remember equipment settings so that the beam is aimed correctly during each session of therapy. The result is a radiation beam of just the right size, of just the right strength, and aimed at just the right spot to cause the most damage to the cancer and the least to the patient.

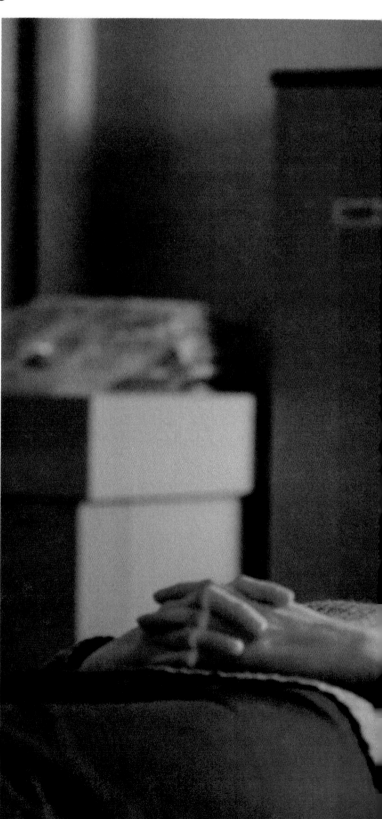

In a demonstration, a physician uses a measuring tape to check the computer's calculation of the distance a radiation simulator beam is to travel. The red spots and line, projected from lasers mounted in the walls and ceiling, serve as reference marks for positioning a patient accurately in the X-ray beam (page 132).

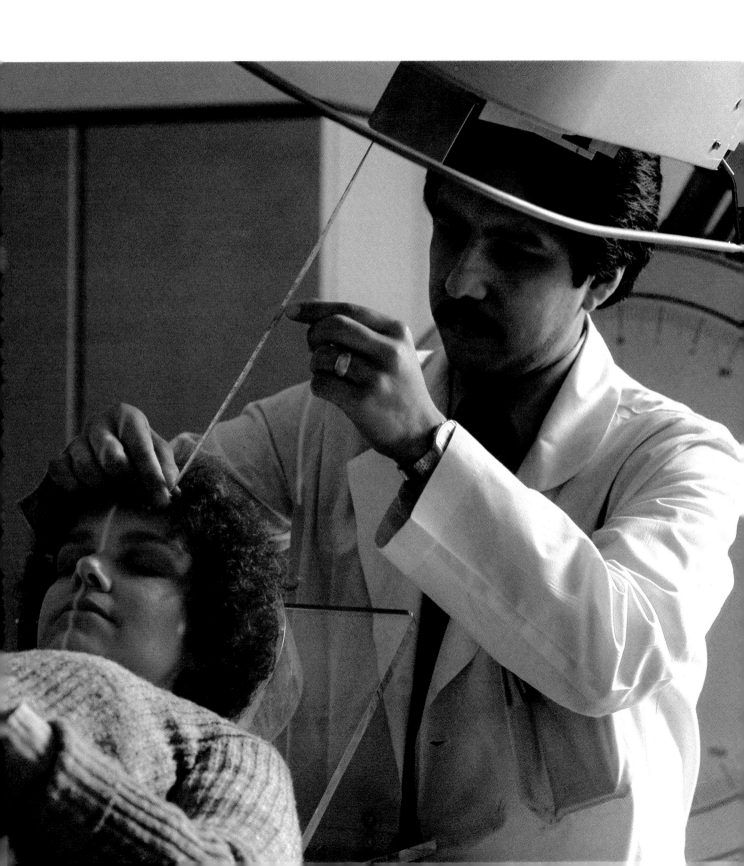

Taking aim at a tumor

Safe and effective radiation therapy demands faultless marksmanship; miss the target, and the patient, not the tumor, may be injured. To be certain of a direct hit, radiation therapists first of all help the patient hold very still, so that he cannot accidentally shift the target out of the treatment beam. But they also refine their aim with practice shots of a weak beam from an X-ray simulator.

Occasionally a patient must be completely immobilized—in the treatment of leukemia, the entire spinal column may be irradiated, and the patient is mummified in a plaster cast. More often, tumors treated with radiation beams are relatively small. Consequently, only part of the body must be kept still. A custom-fitted cradle or a partial cast may be molded to support the part of the body that is targeted for radiation.

With such aids provided, the exact position for treatment is determined with the radiation simulator. This machine is in every essential respect, even to the control room, identical to the equipment used for treatment—save for one crucial exception. Instead of a powerful source of radiation, the simulator contains a low-powered X-ray unit with a beam shaped like those for treatment. Aiming the simulator is exactly like aiming the treatment machine, but no harm is done to healthy tissue.

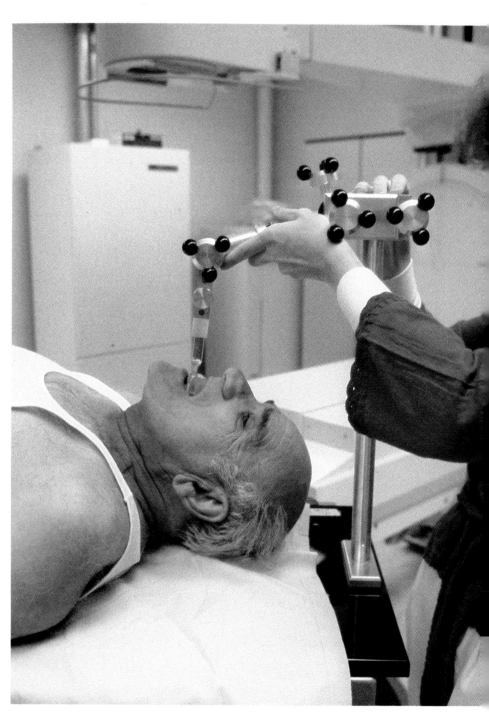

Biting on a custom-fitted mouthpiece, a patient with cancer of the larynx is readied by a technician for the radiation simulator (background). The mouthpiece, attached to a mechanical arm that can be locked in any position, immobilizes the patient's head in the correct position during simulation and in exactly the same position later, during treatment.

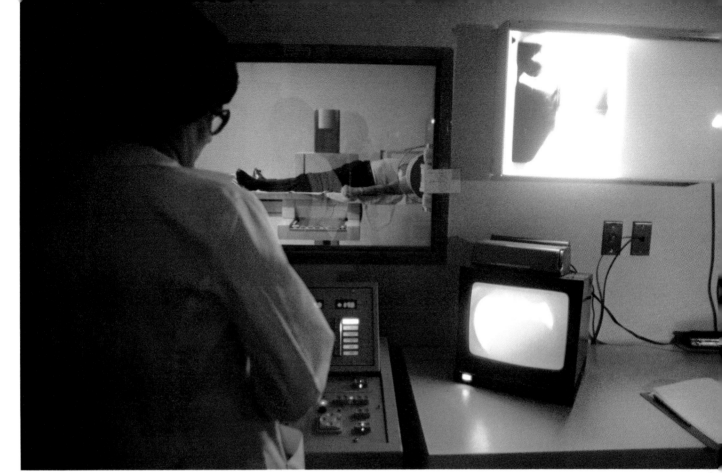

In the control room, a therapist studies a
televised X-ray of her patient as he lies on a
table in the beam of the simulator. Using
the console in front of her to move the table,
she centers the tumor in the beam,
adjusts the simulator angle, then enters the
settings in the computer. The simulator
records a picture of the televised image.

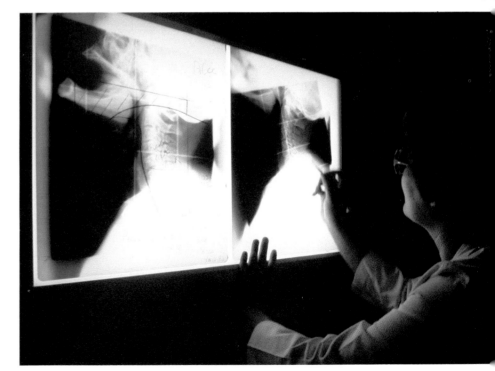

Her marking pencil poised above the
X-ray picture made by the simulator, the
radiation therapist starts to map the
treatment area. To her left, an X-ray that
was taken when the tumor was larger shows
the location of an earlier treatment zone.

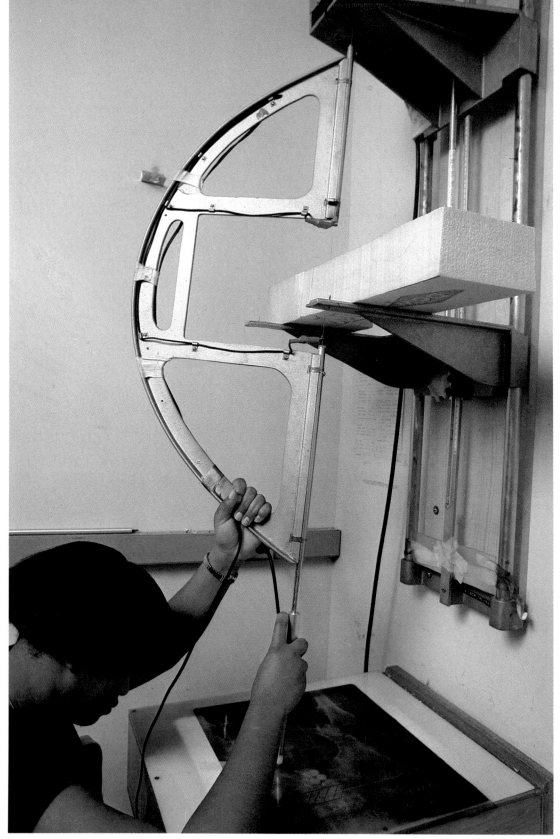

Using a special tool that carves foam plastic with an electrically heated wire, a technician traces the area that needs to be shielded during treatment, following a radiologist's marks on a simulator X-ray on the table. The hole thus cut in the foam plastic is then used as a mold for casting a lead shield.

A foundry in a hospital

The smell of molten metal and the shriek of an electric saw identify an unexpected facet of radiation therapy. The sounds and smells come from the mold shop, a small factory that turns out lead shields and plaster casts to guarantee safe treatments. After treatment has been plotted on a simulator's X-ray picture *(page 113),* the picture becomes a guide *(left)* for carving molds and casting shields. A plaster cast *(overleaf)* may be used to shape a lead-foil mask as protection against the weak radiation applied to skin cancer, as an aid for planning treatment *(page 118)* or simply to help keep a patient still.

Often, one set of radiation shields or a single cast is enough for each patient. But as treatment changes, the mold shop must alter its work or, in some instances, start all over.

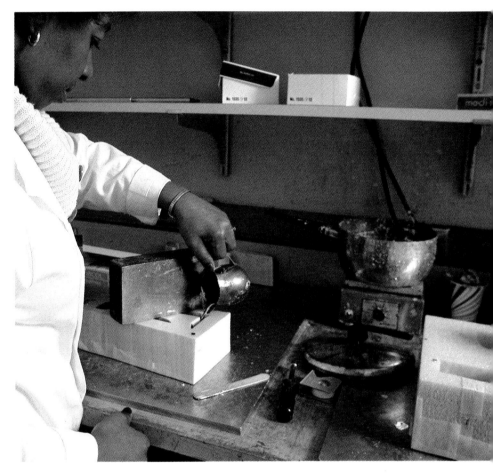

Molten lead alloy, heated in a kitchen pot on a hot plate, is poured into a plastic foam mold. A brick of solid metal anchors the featherweight mold during the pour.

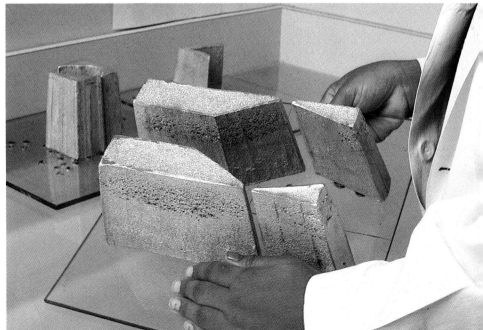

Shiny lead shields, fresh out of the mold, are bolted to a thick plate of clear plastic. When the plate is placed in a radiation beam, the shields protect healthy parts of the patient's body from rays.

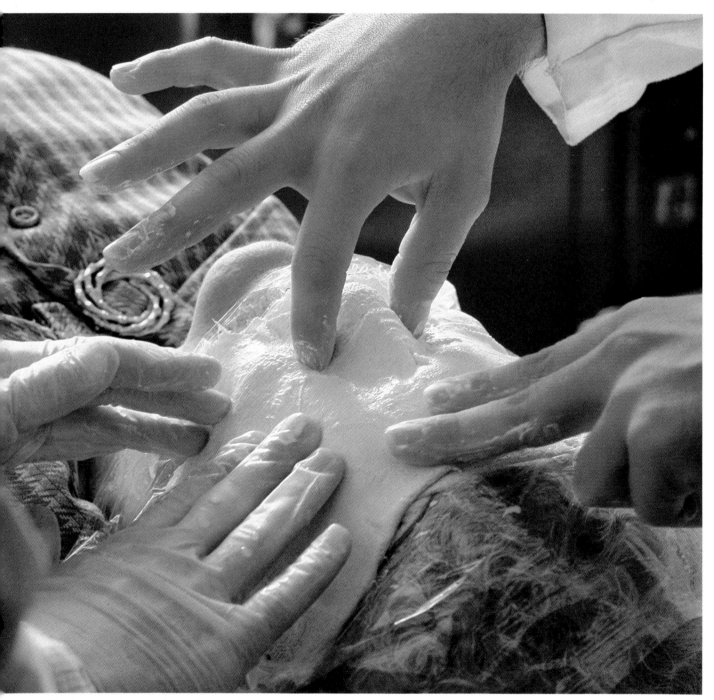

*Mold-shop workers press wet, plaster-laden gauze onto the face of
a woman with skin cancer on her lower eyelid. After the plaster
sets, the cast is lifted from her face to mold a lead-foil mask about
one fifth of an inch thick, which she will wear during treatment.
The radiation goes through a hole cut in it to expose her cancer.*

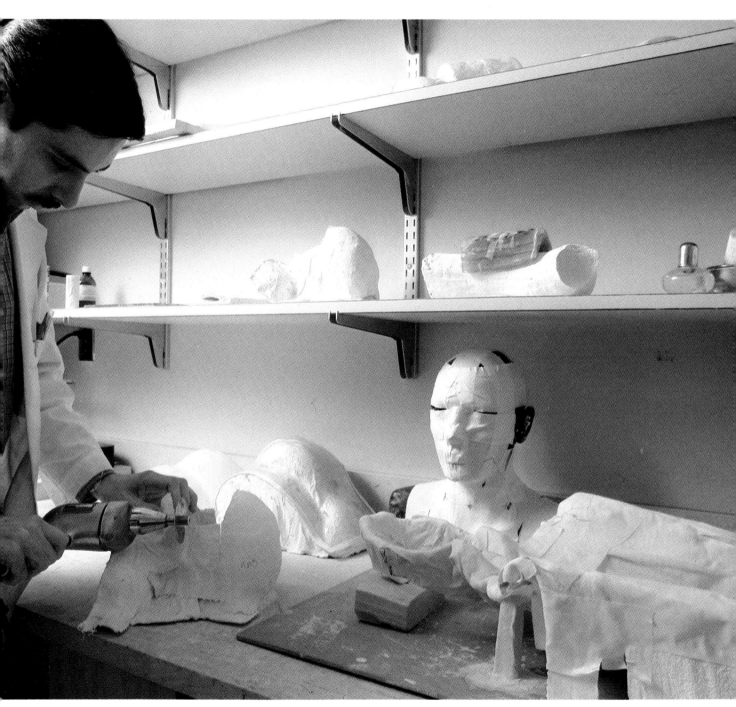

*Working in a clutter of molds and casts, a technician adjusts
the opening in a child's head cast to enlarge the area that will be
irradiated during treatment for a brain tumor. The radiation
must reach the body directly, unimpeded by the plaster, which
would change the path of the beam slightly.*

Dry run on a computer

The final check on radiation planning requires a look deep inside the patient's body to see what the beam of radiation will hit—and how hard. There is no risk to the patient; indeed, he is never present. The entire procedure takes place in a computer.

This computerized dry run begins with a narrow cast of the patient's body contour, made by molding a strip of plaster-laden gauze around him at the tumor location. From this cast, an outline representing a cross section of the patient's body is drawn *(right)*. This outline is fed into the computer, and the computer is instructed to fire simulated bursts of radiation at the tumor from each planned angle of treatment.

Instantly the computer displays a set of lines, resembling contour lines of altitude on a topographical map, that show the intensity of radiation at every point struck by the beam. Bombarding the cancer from several directions multiplies the impact on the tumor while minimizing the amount of radiation penetrating adjacent tissues.

Working from a plaster cast, technicians outline a cross section of a cancer patient's body on graph paper. The doctor then draws in the lead shields that will protect healthy parts of the body and, from recent X-rays, draws the tumor and nearby organs.

With a stylus connected by a cable to the computer, a technician
meticulously traces a body cross section like the one being
drawn at left. As he follows the lines, the computer displays its
copy on the screen to his left. The computer then adds to the
cross section display its calculations of the directions and the
intensities of the planned radiation beams.

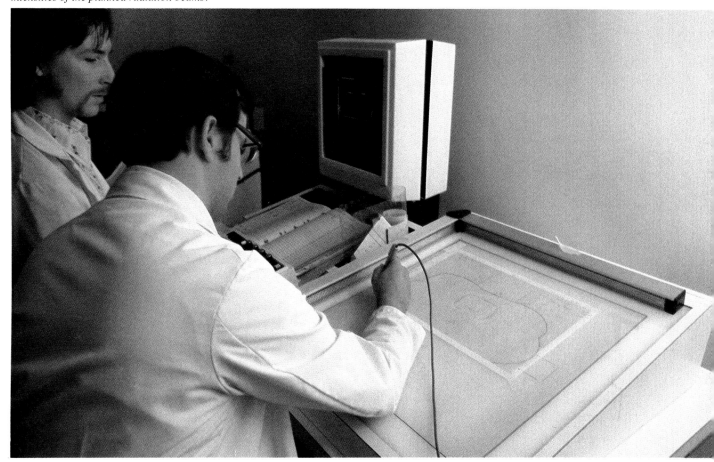

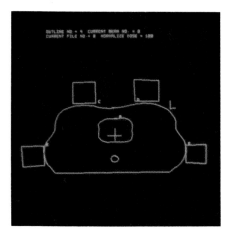

*A patient's spine (circle) and above it an
esophageal tumor appear in cross section in
his torso. The cross marks the beam
center; square shapes are lead shields.*

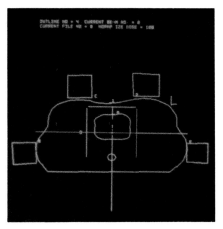

*Beams from the sides and above strike
the tumor—one beam penetrating the spine.
The horizontal line above the tumor and
vertical lines at the sides mark beam widths.*

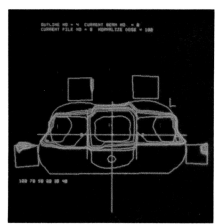

*The tumor outline (center) is surrounded
by contours of radiation intensity. The inner
area gets full strength, the outer ones
lesser percentages listed below the image.*

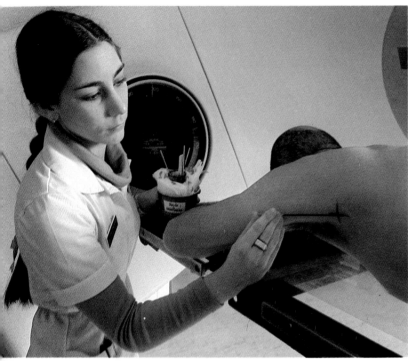

Just before treatment begins, a technician darkens a cross
that will be aligned with laser beams from the walls and ceiling to
position the patient and aim the huge X-ray machine. The
circular scale beyond the patient's head indicates the beam angle.

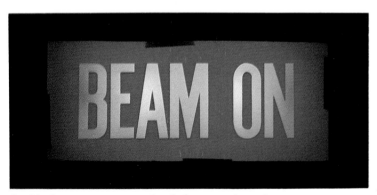

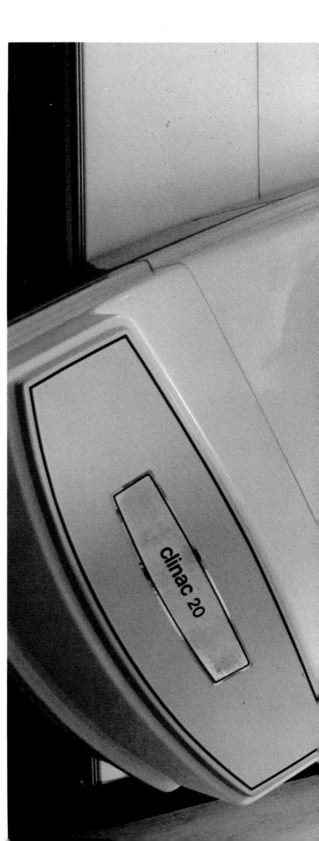

Outside the treatment room a sign flashes a warning to keep
hospital staff away from the dangerous radiation while a
patient is treated. Inside, the scene is like the one at right,
photographed just seconds before the sign flashed on. The
patient lies motionless and alone as the hospital's most powerful
machine, a shield fastened in its muzzle, blasts his cancer.

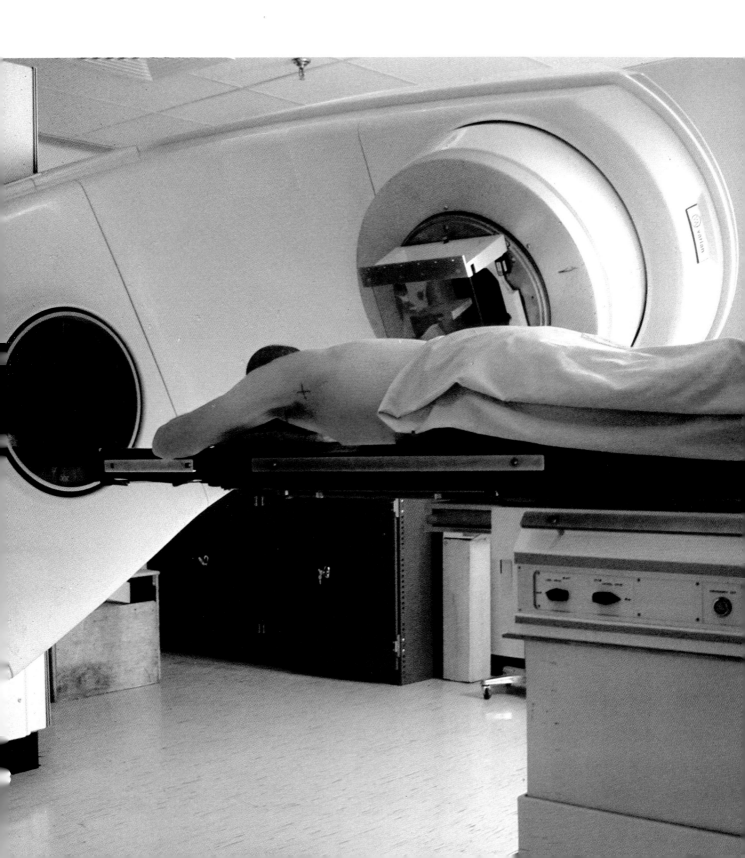

CHAPTER 5

A dream come true: cures that work

Where to go for the best treatment
Weighing options for surgery
How much breast surgery is necessary?
Aid—and danger—from rays
The eerie experience of radiation treatment
Poisoning cancer with chemicals
Far-out ideas that may work

"I was bathing Bradley, my two-year-old son," wrote Sue Cody of Memphis, "when I noticed little blue, bruise-like spots on his back and legs." Bradley was an active boy, so bruises were nothing new. What was new was the number of them. "There were so many of these little dark areas," she said, "that I called the pediatrician, and made an appointment for the following Monday." The day of the visit to the doctor, she recalled, "my world fell apart."

On that dreary October day she learned her son had a form of cancer of the blood—acute lymphocytic leukemia. Small bruises can be a sign of the disease, indicating that the blood's clotting cells, the platelets, are not plentiful enough to prevent slightly injured tissue from bleeding internally.

"I had heard of leukemia," she said, "and I knew it was fatal. That's all I could think of—my two-year-old son would die." He did not. His doctors gave him massive doses of anticancer drugs, compounds with jaw-breaking names such as daunomycin, cyclophosphamide, prednisone, methotrexate and vincristine. Then, to destroy any malignant cells that might have escaped the drug assault, his doctors bombarded him with cancer-killing radiation.

Eleven years later, young Bradley was very much alive, a boisterous, cancer-free 13-year-old. He had conquered the disease and could expect to live a normal life span.

Bradley was no freak case. The reason his disease went away was not that his body overcame it unaided; such spontaneous remission occurs in perhaps one case in 100,000. Rather, Bradley's survival is testimony to the slow, steady progress that has been made in treating cancer. In the 1940s, effective therapy for acute lymphocytic leukemia was unknown, and virtually no one with the disease survived a year past diagnosis. By the 1980s, thanks to the discovery of drugs such as those given Bradley and to the more skillful use of radiation, more than half of the children who contract this form of leukemia live five years or longer after diagnosis.

Survival for five years is generally considered to be a cure. After five years there is only a 1-in-10 chance of relapse; after 10 years, the chance of relapse is virtually nil.

What is true of acute lymphocytic leukemia is true for many other kinds of cancer: Treatment has dramatically improved. Doctors have perfected their oldest anticancer weapon, surgery, so that huge tumors, previously unapproachable, can be removed. Modern radiation treatments exterminate malignant cells by disturbing their biological processes—leaving healthy cells, just millimeters away, little affected. And new classes of drugs, used singly or in combinations, poison cancer cells without killing the patient. Increasingly all three kinds of treatment are used in combination. And this three-pronged attack may eventually become four-pronged. Immunotherapy, the use of substances that stimulate the body's natural defenses to fight the disease, has shown promise in some clinical trials.

Progress in treating 12 types of cancer—two kinds of leukemia, four lymph cancers, and certain cancers of the bone, head and neck, kidney, uterus, testes, and ovaries— has been so great that they are now considered curable by

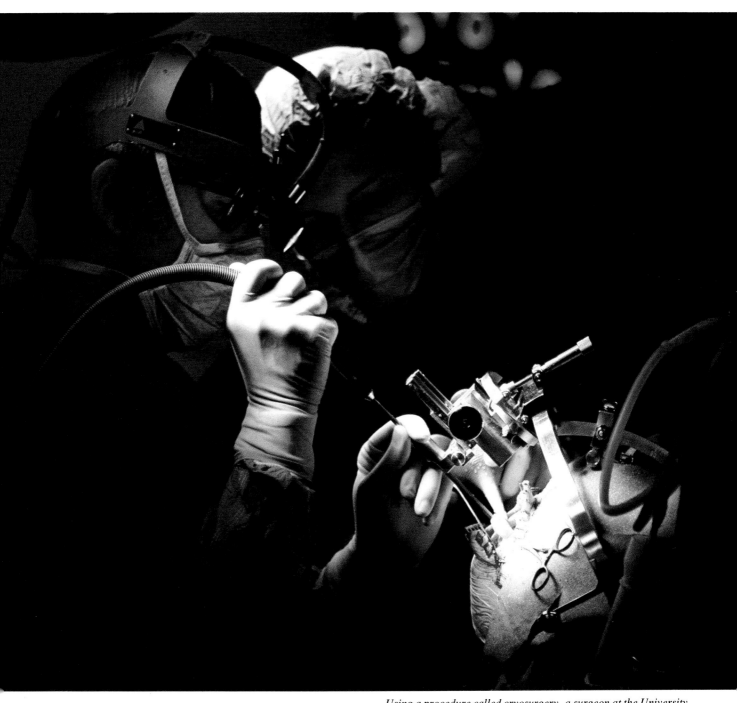

Using a procedure called cryosurgery, a surgeon at the University of California at Los Angeles directs a stream of –320° F. liquid nitrogen into a patient's pituitary-gland cancer. Repeated freezing and thawing kills the malignant cells during the half-hour operation, and after two or three weeks they disappear.

conventional therapies. Relatively little progress has been made in treating the most deadly form of the disease, lung cancer. But if deaths from this largely preventable disease were eliminated from the statistics, the five-year survival rate in the United States for 1981—excluding easily cured skin and uterine cancers—would jump from just above 40 per cent to around 60 per cent.

"I often wonder if we aren't overstressing the fact that we can't 'cure' more cancer patients," said Dr. Michael Friedman of the University of California's Cancer Research Institute. "I don't know of many other major diseases of the adult world that are cured. Most adult chronic diseases we treat are palliated for the life of the patient. As far as I know, no one has ever been really cured of diabetes mellitus or chronic obstructive pulmonary disease or coronary artery disease." A 26-year-old patient echoed that optimism: "No one wants to get cancer, but at least I have a curable disease."

Where to go for the best treatment

For the greatest chance of cure, a cancer patient must get the right treatment, and get it immediately. The first shot at the disease may be the only good shot. Delay permits cancer cells to spread throughout the body so that they can elude complete control.

Equally important is the kind of treatment. Even treatment begun at the first sign of disease will let slip that first crucial opportunity for cure if the measures taken are ill chosen or ill applied. For handling cancer, more than for treating most other diseases, not all doctors and not all hospitals are equal.

First-rate cancer treatment is seldom provided by a single physician, however competent he may be. It requires a small army of specialists in cancer surgery, radiation and drugs— at the University of Alabama Medical Center in Birmingham, a typical cancer patient has three or more physicians actively engaged in his case. What is more, to achieve the best results, these specialists must have at hand enormous medical resources—costly equipment, teams of technicians and specialized know-how that usually are found only at large hospitals and university medical centers.

As a rule, family physicians lack the special training need-

How early diagnosis improves the odds

Proof that early detection of cancer can make the difference between life and death is contained in cure rates for nine common types *(right)* that affect particular organs. For each type, the graph contrasts the percentages of American patients surviving five years or longer after diagnosis, according to the extent to which a cancer has spread. Three stages of spreading are indicated. The least is a single small tumor localized within the organ in which it began. More serious is cancer that has spread beyond its origin to other tissue in the same organ, to nearby connective tissue or to adjacent lymph nodes. Most dangerous is cancer spread to other organs or distant parts of the body.

In all except the deadliest of the malignancies listed—lung cancer—detection while tumors are localized *(green)* brings better than a 50-50 chance of cure. And even for lung cancer, such early diagnosis more than triples the survival rate.

In some types of cancer—tumors of the breast, lower intestine and prostate gland—slight spreading *(blue)* lessens the cure rate only somewhat. In these types, the standard treatment includes surgery that removes enough tissue to eliminate not only the original tumor but also nearby tissue that may harbor undetected cancer cells. But for any of the nine, delay in diagnosis until malignancy has spread beyond nearby tissue into other organs or to remote parts of the body *(red)* makes the odds of survival at best 1 in 5.

ed to treat cancer. But they frequently perform one of the most important roles in the entire process—referring patients to doctors who do specialize in the disease. In most instances the specialist will then assume overall responsibility for the case; usually the family physician will remain involved, monitoring the patient's general health and serving as liaison between the patient and the specialists. This referral system is followed almost everywhere. In some countries that have comprehensive governmental systems of medical care, such as Great Britain, the choice of specialists may be more limited than in the United States or West Germany— the patient is generally referred only to one of the specific cancer physicians with whom the family doctor is enrolled in the national health scheme. This distinction between countries, however, is often more theoretical than real.

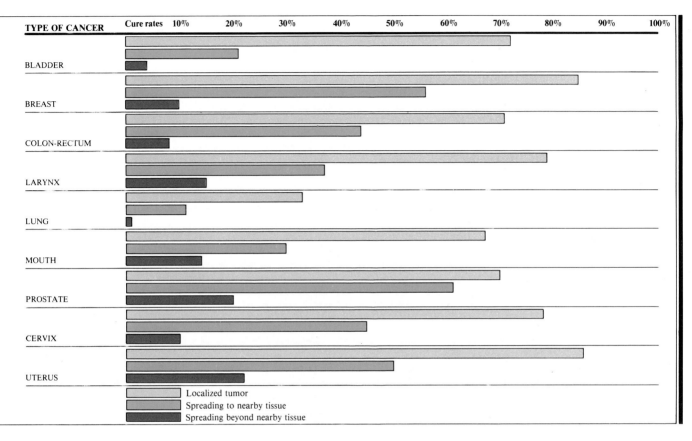

TYPE OF CANCER	Cure rates	10%	20%	30%	40%	50%	60%	70%	80%	90%	100%
BLADDER											
BREAST											
COLON-RECTUM											
LARYNX											
LUNG											
MOUTH											
PROSTATE											
CERVIX											
UTERUS											

Localized tumor
Spreading to nearby tissue
Spreading beyond nearby tissue

In almost any country, the patient has more control over his care than he may realize—or choose to exert. He need not accept a specialist to whom he is referred, and he owes it to himself to make certain that he gets into the hands of a competent practitioner skilled in treating his ailment.

Although the variety of cancer physicians is confusingly large, surgeons are the usual choice except in cases of leukemia, many lymph cancers and inoperable lung malignancies; these cancers are most often handled by drug or radiation specialists. Surgeons normally perform the definitive cancer diagnosis—the surgical biopsy *(pages 86-91)*.

Most surgeons themselves specialize, operating only on particular organs or bodily systems. Thus an individual with a suspected cancer of the colon likely would be referred to a colon and rectal surgeon, a person with possible bladder or kidney cancer to a urologist or urological surgeon, a woman with ovarian cancer to a gynecological surgeon, and a person with possible lung cancer to a thoracic, or chest, surgeon. Because these subspecialists have extra schooling in their chosen fields, they are generally better qualified to treat certain cancers than either family doctors or general surgeons—doctors trained to operate on many parts of the body, but particularly on the abdominal region. Yet because cancer surgery is so prevalent, some general surgeons devote a high proportion of their practice to it. In addition, increasing numbers of general surgeons have added postgraduate training in oncology, the treatment of cancer, to their credentials.

A potential patient can sometimes learn the details of a physician's specialized training by telephone. The information almost always can be read off the wall of his office.

Hanging there will be one or more certificates, testifying that the doctor has acquired a minimum number of years of postgraduate training in a particular field and has passed written and oral examinations relating to it. In the United States these certificates are issued by so-called boards, such as the American Board of Colon & Rectal Surgery, the American Board of Obstetrics & Gynecology and the American Board of Urology. Most other Western countries do not have certification boards as such; a doctor's specialty certificate will have been issued by the university where he trained.

The fact that a physician has been certified in a specialty is one indication of his standing in the medical community. However, many older doctors of superior competence acquired their skills before such formal training was common, and thus may not be certified. Hospital associations are another clue. A good specialist usually has staff privileges at a university medical center or several community hospitals; that is, he is allowed to treat patients there on a regular basis.

A third factor to consider in assessing a specialist is his familiarity with the specific procedure proposed—in the case of a surgeon, how often he performs a particular operation. This information can be acquired only by asking, but the patient has a right to know. The answer must be evaluated in the context of some background information, for certain procedures are obviously more common than others.

For one common cancer often referred to general surgeons—breast cancer—the following figure can be used for comparison: At a leading American hospital, the Memorial Sloan-Kettering Cancer Center in New York, a general surgeon who does virtually nothing but breast-cancer operations performs breast surgery about 10 times a week. For a rarer form, such as liver cancer, an expert general surgeon at Sloan-Kettering performs three operations a week. At even a first-class community hospital such as Fairfax Hospital in northern Virginia, the average is much lower; an expert general surgeon there does about three operations a month for breast cancer and may do liver surgery only twice a year.

The choice of specialist for primary cancer care generally determines where that care will be provided. Most local surgeons operate only in nearby community hospitals. Many of these facilities are well equipped for cancer treatment. But for the most elaborate care, a patient must go to one of the large regional facilities, university medical centers or special institutes. They can afford the newest diagnostic and therapeutic equipment, and can attract the best and brightest doctors in the field. As centers of research and treatment, they often test recently devised therapies, using experimental drugs or new combinations of drugs, surgery and radiation.

In 1971 the National Cancer Institute (NCI) began to single out comprehensive cancer centers in many American cities for special support by the federal government. Italy has the Istituto Nazionale Tumori in Milan, France the Hôpital Saint-Antoine in Paris and the Institute Gustave-Roussy in Villejuif, Belgium the Institute Jules Bordet in Brussels, Japan the National Cancer Center in Tokyo, Canada the Ontario Cancer Foundation in Windsor. In the Soviet Union the Cancer Research Center in Moscow is the nation's main cancer hospital, but there are more than 250 specialized cancer facilities throughout the country.

Although such cancer centers offer treatment that may be significantly better than that available in a community hospital, their disadvantages must also be considered. For many people these facilities are far from home, and some patients find them large and impersonal.

No matter which doctor and hospital are selected, the patient must be an active participant in the process. "It hasn't been scientifically proven," said Dr. Paul K. Hamilton, former head of the Oncology Unit at the Presbyterian Medical Center in Denver, Colorado, "but my experience is that a patient who assumes responsibility for his or her own healing and health, and who has a quality relationship with the physician, is more cooperative, requires less medication for pain or sleep, and shows more favorable response to treatment."

The patient—or his family—must be prepared to ask questions of his doctors, to demand explanations of the procedures and therapies that are proposed. "People tend to hold physicians in awe," wrote Drs. Harold Glucksberg and Jack W. Singer of the Fred Hutchinson Cancer Research Center in Seattle, Washington. "It is difficult for the patient to think of his rights or needs, especially when he has cancer and is crying out for help. However, there are many occasions,'' the doctors continued, ''when you, the patient, need to stand up for your own interests.''

Weighing options for surgery

Nowhere is the patient's participation more important than in the treatment that in half of all cancer cases is the first form of therapy—surgery. Because the operation occasionally can be debilitating and disfiguring, it is doubly important to understand the procedure that is proposed. Write down questions beforehand and take notes as they are answered. Demand to know what percentage of patients who have had similar surgery have lived five years or longer. Ask whether other treatments might offer comparable results. Find out how disabling and disfiguring the surgery is likely to be. Ask about the risk of death or permanent disability from the operation or its complications. It is very helpful to have a family member or friend present during this discussion; he may remember questions or recall information otherwise missed.

Cancer surgery should not be delayed but it is rarely emergency surgery. ''It does not have to be done in a matter of hours or even days,'' noted Drs. Glucksberg and Singer. ''You have time to see another surgeon for a second opinion. If it does nothing else, a second opinion will give you more confidence in your surgeon.'' Most of the time it does just that: In one Boston survey of 1,591 patients who sought second opinions in surgery, 89 per cent received second opinions that agreed with the first.

Because surgery aims to cut out all of the malignant cells in one swoop, in many instances it offers the best chance of cure—each year, more cancer patients are cured by surgery than by radiation and drugs combined.

''If one were to restrict oneself to a single weapon,'' stated the French cancer specialist Dr. Lucien Israël, ''one would have to choose surgery.'' Indeed, surgery is medicine's oldest cancer weapon. Hippocrates, the father of medicine, wrote of removing cancerous breasts in the Fourth Century B.C., and the procedure was not new then. The great Greek physician is also the author of the Hippocratic Oath, which forswears harm to a patient. Yet for millennia surgical efforts often did more harm than good. Anesthesia and antiseptic techniques were essentially unknown; patients who survived the trauma of an operation generally died from infection.

By the late 19th Century, the introduction of anesthesia and antiseptic surgery enabled a Viennese physician, Theodor Billroth, to operate successfully on patients with cancers of the stomach and intestines. In the 1890s Dr. William Halstead, Professor of Surgery at The Johns Hopkins University in Baltimore, developed surgical techniques, still known by his name, that became standard for treating breast cancer. Since Dr. Halstead's time the steady improvement of instruments and techniques has brought virtually every portion of the human body within the surgeon's reach. Today tumors are not only cut out by scalpels but are destroyed by powerful electrical currents, burned away by concentrated light beams from lasers, dissolved by strong chemical agents or frozen by the −320° F. chill of liquid nitrogen. Advances in anesthesia permit patients to be kept safely unconscious for operations that can last up to 15 hours. Blood transfusions control life-threatening shock. Antibiotics inhibit postoperative infection. And, perhaps most remarkably, the development in the 1950s of the heart-lung machine has permitted doctors to operate on those critical organs while the device breathes and pumps blood for the anesthetized patient.

A drastic cure for intestinal cancer

The most common of the cancers requiring extensive surgery are those striking the breast, colon or rectum. The surgery involved also has extraordinary impact on many patients, for it may entail alteration of body structures that seems drastic in prospect, though much less so in retrospect.

''I felt so well,'' wrote New York author and public relations executive Letitia Baldrige, that ''I couldn't come to grips with the fact that I had cancer.'' She had just been told that she had a dark mass in her colon, almost certainly malignant. Her internist sent her immediately to a surgeon, John Whitsell at New York Hospital-Cornell Medical Center.

There, Dr. Whitsell explained step by step what he planned to do. First, he would cut off a piece of the dark mass—perform a biopsy—to determine beyond question whether the growth was malignant. If it was, he said, "we will have to go in and remove that large mass in the colon."

Such an operation, Dr. Whitsell continued, would take one of two forms. If the malignancy was located above the rectum, the growth could be cut out and the two cut ends of the bowel reconnected. If the rectum was involved, however, it would have to be removed and a new pathway created. That pathway, the doctor explained, was a colostomy—a permanent opening for the intestine in the lower abdominal wall.

If a colostomy proved necessary, body wastes would pass through the opening and be collected in a disposable plastic pouch. "That, I felt sure, was not going to happen," recalled the patient. But it did. "I resolved simply to accept the plastic bag," she said. "When you consider the alternative, wearing it doesn't mean a blasted thing. I'd had a tumor the size of a small grapefruit; it had to go. Now it *was* gone and I was still here." A week after leaving the hospital, she flew to Miami for a speaking engagement. Within a month, she said, "I was back on my usual 15-hour treadmill."

Letitia Baldrige was one of more than 100,000 Americans who are stricken with colo-rectal cancer each year. More than half undergo colostomies. Thanks largely to this

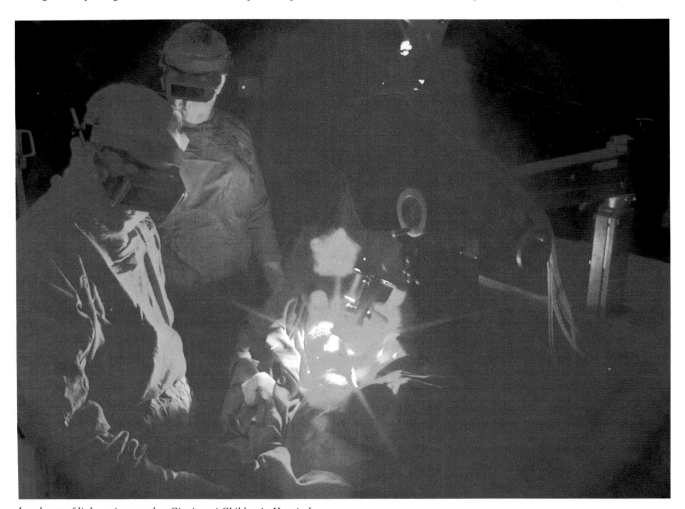

In a burst of light so intense that Cincinnati Children's Hospital surgeons avert their shielded eyes, a laser beam boils away cancerous cells on a woman's leg. This substitute for a scalpel, developed in the 1950s, concentrates enormous heat and power in a tight beam of amplified light waves. The treatment is usually painless, and healthy cells soon grow over the burned area.

operation, about 70 per cent of patients undergoing surgery for early colo-rectal cancer survive the first five years.

Today many cancers once curable only with colostomy can be treated by less drastic procedures. This change has come about since the invention in the Soviet Union of a staple gun, called an end-to-end anastomosis stapler, that fastens together the cut ends of the colon with a double circle of stainless-steel staples, each one fifth of an inch long. The stapler can reach all around the colon, inside the narrow confines of the pelvic area, much more readily than a surgeon's hands. It can securely reattach the colon and rectum even when only a small portion of the rectum remains intact. Such reattachment leaves the patient with a more or less normal intestinal system, eliminating the need for the colostomy and pouch. At the Cleveland Clinic, reported its Chairman of Colo-rectal Surgery, Dr. Victor W. Fazio, colostomies are "down by at least a third" because of the stapler.

How much breast surgery is necessary?

For breast cancer, as for malignancies of the colon or rectum, surgery is commonly the treatment. About 111,000 new cases of breast cancer are diagnosed each year in the United States; in more than 90,000 of those, women have the breast removed—a mastectomy. In England more than 20,000 mastectomies are performed each year, in France about the same number, in Japan nearly 8,000.

Despite the heartening testimonials of many famous women who have had mastectomies—including former First Lady Betty Ford and the former Vice President's wife, Happy Rockefeller—these operations have aroused extensive controversy. Many of them apply the original Halstead procedure, which requires removal not only of the breast but also of underlying chest muscle and underarm lymph nodes, which spread cancer. The effect on body shape is considerable, and arm movement may be permanently restricted. Several new therapies promise at least to reduce the impact of breast-cancer treatment and, if the cancer is caught early, possibly even to eliminate the need for breast removal.

Since 1951 large-scale studies in many countries have compared the survival rates obtained by the Halstead mastec-

tomy with those achieved by the less extensive modified radical mastectomy, in which the breast and lymph nodes are removed but underlying chest muscles are left intact. Virtually without exception, the studies showed no significant advantage for the Halstead mastectomy.

These findings led a panel on breast cancer, convened by the National Cancer Institute in 1979, to recommend that the Halstead mastectomy be replaced by the modified procedure as the standard breast-cancer treatment in the United States.

Several preliminary studies have indicated that even the modified mastectomy can sometimes be avoided. One procedure—lumpectomy—differs little from the simple diagnostic biopsy. In that operation only the detectable lumps and a small portion of adjacent tissue are removed from a cancerous breast. Then the afflicted breast is treated with radiation. In one study of this method, conducted by Dr. Sackari Mustakallio of Helsinki, 702 women with breast tumors were reviewed. With the exception of only one group—women 65 or older with large tumors—lumpectomy followed by radiation proved more effective than total breast removal.

Other ongoing breast-cancer studies indicate that drug therapy combined with surgery may improve the overall cure rates. Many of the trials have been too limited to yield convincing evidence, but for one large group of patients—women who have not reached menopause—the results are conclusive. Dr. Gianni Bonnadonna of the Istituto Nazionale per lo Studio e la Cura dei Tumori in Milan studied 189 premenopausal women suffering from breast cancer. They were separated into two study groups: one treated with mastectomies alone, the other with both mastectomies and drug therapy. After five years, 69.4 per cent of the women treated with mastectomies and drugs were alive, compared with 44.3 per cent of those who had had mastectomies alone.

For any kind of cancer, the trend is toward such combination treatment. Surgery alone is used only for a few types of easily cured skin cancers and for early malignancies confined to a single part of the body. Surgery often is combined with drugs in treating advanced cancers of the stomach, for a bone cancer known as osteogenic sarcoma, and for a dangerous skin cancer called malignant melanoma. Surgery is teamed with radiation for many cancers of the cervix, uterus, kidneys, head and neck, tongue, colon, lung and rectum, and also for some bladder cancers and many so-called soft-tissue sarcomas. Surgery occasionally is followed by both radiation and chemotherapy not only for breast and a few colon and rectal cancers but also for cancers of the liver, pancreas and ovaries; some cancers of the lymph systems and testes; some bone and brain tumors; and almost all cases of Wilms' tumor, a childhood kidney cancer.

Aid—and danger—from rays

The increased use of radiation stems from tremendous strides in techniques and equipment. Doctors today have more powerful and more precise machines than ever before. Experience has taught them which types of cancer respond to radiotherapy, and which do not. Further, they know when to give radiation treatment, and in what doses, in order to cause most damage to the tumor and least harm to the patient. "We are looking at the possibility," said Dr. DeVita of NCI, "that in 15 to 20 years cancer patients will not only live longer, but live intact. That means less surgery and more of something else for local disease. That something else is radiotherapy."

The two forms of radiation therapy still most commonly used were discovered within three years of each other, nearly a century ago. One is the X-rays used for diagnosis, discovered by Wilhelm Conrad Roentgen in Würzburg in 1895. The other was found by Marie and Pierre Curie in Paris. The Curies observed rays emanating from pitchblende ores; they traced the rays' origin to a previously unknown element in the ore, radium. Its rays, like X-rays, could penetrate cloth and flesh but were at least partially blocked by denser substances such as metal and bone, and they could be used to make shadow pictures on photographic film.

The emanations from radium were given the name gamma rays. Soon the same rays were detected arising in other radioactive elements. It also became clear that gamma rays and X-rays are essentially identical: streams of electromagnetic energy like light or radio waves but with wavelengths 10,000 times shorter than the shortest visible light waves. The difference lies in their sources. X-rays are generated by electronic vacuum tubes; gamma rays by the disintegration of the nuclei, or cores, within atoms.

The early experimenters with X-rays and gamma rays quickly realized that both could be harmful. Painful, burn-like sores appeared on skin exposed repeatedly to the rays. These damaging effects suggested to turn-of-the-century physicians that the rays might be used to burn out cancerous growths. One of the first to whom this thought occurred was an experimenter named E. H. Grubbe.

In 1896 Grubbe, who had been working with X-rays in his Chicago laboratory, grew alarmed when a painful skin condition erupted on his left hand. He went to a doctor, named J. E. Gillman, who treated him for dermatitis. It was concluded that the skin condition might be related to Grubbe's X-ray work. Next, they asked themselves a logical question: If X-rays could harm normal skin cells, could they also harm abnormal growths? Dr. Gillman then asked Grubbe to test the hypothesis on one of his patients, a woman with incurable breast cancer. Grubbe agreed. The results of the experiment have been lost to history. But it is almost certain that the amounts of radiation delivered to the woman's tumor would have been insufficient to produce any significant improvement. Nevertheless, Grubbe is generally recognized as the first to treat a cancer patient with radiation.

Radium was first used on cancer in 1901, by Henri Alexandre Danlos, a dermatologist in Paris who treated a patient with skin cancer by applying a radium mixture to the skin.

These intrepid pioneers were taking shots in the dark. But hard evidence that radiation could indeed help battle cancer soon came from tests on animals. In France in 1906 Jean Bergonie and Louis Tribondeau irradiated rat tissues and found that X-rays not only harm living cells but damage certain kinds more than others. The most vulnerable tissues proved to be those containing rapidly multiplying cells. Thus X-rays or gamma rays passing into the body strike selectively at a cancer, killing off many of its proliferating cells while causing much less harm to other tissues they hit.

Soon safe dosage schemes were worked out, and both radium and X-rays were put to work treating cancer. Meanwhile, physicists delving into the ultimate nature of matter by

In a scene he painted himself, Dr. Georges Chicotot times X-ray treatment of a cancerous breast at the Hôpital Broca in Paris in 1908, three years after radiation was first used to treat cancer in France. But why the top hat? Dr. Chicotot, it turns out, wore it not for vanity's sake but in the misguided belief that it would protect him from the potentially harmful rays.

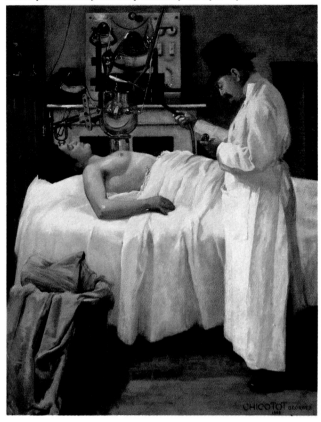

smashing atoms found other rays—streams of minuscule fragments of atoms that were so energetic they had the same—or greater—effect on cancer as X-rays or gamma rays. In fact, until World War II, much of the financial support for this research into nuclear physics was raised by scientists who promised that the very expensive atom-smashing machines they wanted to build would, some day, lead to a cure for cancer. And they have.

Why X-rays, gamma rays and atomic particles are such selective killers of proliferating cancer cells is only partially understood. Apparently the enormous energy carried by the rays is absorbed inordinately by cellular nuclei. Within the nuclei, radiation's effects seem to be concentrated on the master molecules that control multiplication, DNA and RNA *(Chapter 4)*. The radiation produces profound changes in the DNA and RNA, alterations that kill the cell outright, prevent it from dividing—or introduce a subtle change that causes death not to the irradiated cell itself but to its descendants three or four generations later.

The impact on the duplication mechanisms of DNA and RNA helps explain the rays' selective effect on cancer cells. Their DNA and RNA are busier than those of healthy cells and more readily disrupted. The more powerful the rays, the greater the disruption. Greater power—measured by comparison with electrical pressure, or voltage—also brings other advantages. It focuses the rays into a sharper beam, permitting precise aiming that delivers maximum energy to the cancer target. Higher power also makes the rays penetrate deeper into the body, treating tumors that previously had been unreachable. By the 1930s multithousand-volt machines were on the market, more powerful than the gamma rays from radium. By the late 1940s machines were capable of delivering radiation to tumors at many millions of volts.

Today an enormous variety of complex machines and techniques is used to generate radiation for treating cancer: atom-smashing machines such as cyclotrons, other machines called betatrons and linear accelerators, seeds, needles, fluids containing man-made substitutes for scarce radium, and occasionally even nuclear reactors. The kinds of radiation generated are equally varied, including such nuclear particles as neutrons, protons and pions. Most cancer patients, however, receive X-rays—from an electronic tube basically similar to Roentgen's—or gamma rays generated by a betatron or released by an artificial radioactive material such as cobalt 60, gold 198, cesium 137 or phosphorus 32.

More than half of all cancer patients receive some kind of radiation therapy—particularly those with Hodgkin's disease, some head and neck tumors, or lymphosarcoma. For one out of three, it is part of the primary treatment.

In a minority of cases gamma-emitting substances are implanted directly in the nest of cancer cells. Tiny pellets are inserted into the tumor, often through hollow needles or plastic tubes. Alternatively, doctors may implant radioactive pieces of wire or capsules housing liquids. And sometimes liquids are injected directly into a tumor or into tissues surrounding it. The implants occasionally are left in the body permanently, but usually are taken out after one to six days. This method of radioactive implantation—or internal irradiation—often is used to treat cancers of the head and neck, lip and tongue, voice box, cervix, uterus and prostate gland.

The great majority of tumors, however, are either too large, too inaccessible or too widespread to allow for radioactive implants. Instead, the patient is placed in the path of the radiation stream emerging from the source—most of the devices are so big they cannot be moved to point at the patient. Then the stream is released—either by switching on the equipment to generate the radiation or by opening a port so rays that are constantly being produced can stream out.

The eerie experience of radiation treatment

Radiation treatment, whatever the type, is scary: The rays cannot be seen, heard or, in most cases, even felt, but their danger is evident. The technicians who administer the treatment cannot even stay in the room with the patient, but must operate the equipment from enclosed, heavily shielded con-

trol booths. The equipment itself looks frightening. And the aftereffects are unpleasant, though seldom dangerous.

"My fears all came upon me when I saw the corridor," wrote Laurel Lee, a 30-year-old mother of two from Portland, Oregon. She was scheduled to undergo her first radiation treatment for Hodgkin's disease, a cancer of the lymph system that is particularly sensitive to radiation. "Patients," she remembered, "were treated behind lead-lined doors that read: DANGER. KEEP OUT. HIGH RADIATION AREA."

She was ushered through one of the doors. "I was helped onto a table next to a panel of buttons," she recalled. "Arching over me was a hood, looking like a large green praying mantis, with dials of numbers for eyes." The insect-like machine was a simulator, an X-ray device that enables doctors to plot precisely the area to be irradiated. Guided by pictures from the simulator, Laurel Lee's doctors marked her skin with indelible ink to indicate the areas corresponding to the tumors deep inside her body. During the course of her treatment, the marks would serve as the bull's eyes for the radiation. Once the tumors were targeted, shields were

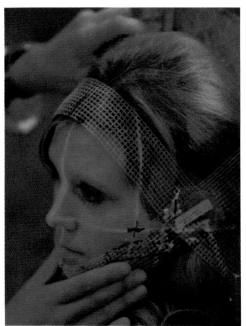

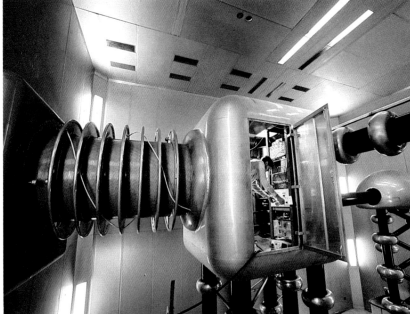

Crossed bands of red laser light are used to line up a powerful beam of neutron atomic particles with its target in this demonstration of brain-cancer treatment at Fermi National Accelerator Laboratory in Batavia, Illinois. The head straps prevent movement while a technician in a shielded booth (right) operates the giant atom smasher that produces neutrons.

custom-made to protect her healthy organs from the rays.

For the actual treatment, her doctors used a betatron machine. ''I was rolled under its girth,'' she recalled. Earplugs were applied because the machine roared as it worked. The therapy took three minutes—an average amount of time.

Like most patients, Laurel Lee reported no sensations during the treatment; some people feel a mild warmth or tingling. But like most, she did suffer nausea and fatigue later. So did Nick Tanis, a film instructor at New York University, also treated for Hodgkin's disease. ''What happens with this stuff,'' he said, ''is that it slowly enervates, it slowly takes away your strength, and you don't know what hit you until all of a sudden you can't get out of bed.''

Other side effects are less common. Some patients lose their hair. Others may find that their skin darkens or reddens, or it becomes tender or itchy, moist or dry. People who receive radiation in the head and neck area or in the upper chest often complain of sore throats, of sores in the mouth or a dry mouth, of difficulty in swallowing or a loss of taste. Some patients irradiated in the lower abdomen become sterile, as do most whose sex organs are irradiated.

Except for sterility, the aftereffects are transient. Nick Tanis got through his treatments and survived the disease. So did Laurel Lee—and so did the healthy baby girl she bore within two months of her radiation therapy.

Poisoning cancer with chemicals

If cancer has spread widely—or if it is a type that infests the entire body, such as cancer of the blood or lymph system—neither radiation nor surgery can be relied on for a cure. Then the newest form of treatment, chemotherapy with cancer-killing drugs, becomes the principal weapon in the battle. Drugs are largely responsible for the remarkable change in outlook for patients with leukemia or Hodgkin's disease—both once sentences of death and now generally curable. In addition, these drugs are increasingly used in combination with surgery or radiation, or both. Drugs are the primary treatment in only about 10 to 15 per cent of all cases, but they are administered at some point in about 25 to 30 per cent.

The search for substances to kill cancer began in antiquity.

Over the centuries, all kinds of materials—snake venom, pokeweed, skunk oil, kerosene, scorpion juice—were used in vain. Paul of Aegina, a Seventh Century Egyptian physician, quoted one colleague's prescription: ''Mix equal parts of burnt river crabs and calamine, and sprinkle or apply the ashes of crabs with cerate.'' Not until the mid-20th Century did scientists discover chemicals that could kill cancer cells without killing the host. In 1942 Dr. Alfred Gilman of the Yale Medical School demonstrated that mechlorethamine, the active ingredient in the deadly chemical-warfare agent known as mustard gas, could produce a dramatic reduction in the size of certain tumors of the lymph glands. Though preliminary, the findings were promising.

Dr. Gilman's tentative research, shrouded in wartime secrecy, received a wholly unexpected and accidental boost the following year. At about 7:30 p.m. on December 2, 1943, German bombers struck a convoy of Allied ships anchored in the harbor of Bari, Italy. The cargo of one of the stricken ships, the U.S.S. John Harvey, included more than 100 tons of poisonous mustard gas. When the bombs hit, the containers ruptured, spilling the noxious chemical into the harbor. Within a month, 83 men plucked from the poisoned waters had died from exposure to the substance.

Autopsies revealed a curious characteristic: blood samples taken from the victims contained markedly fewer white blood cells than normal. White blood cells, which help fight infections, are among the body's most rapidly dividing cells. If mechlorethamine could destroy those cells, reasoned a U.S. Navy doctor named Peter Alexander, might the chemical also kill rapidly dividing malignant cells?

Dr. Alexander reported his findings and his hypotheses to Dr. C. P. Rhodes in New York, then serving as an expert on chemical warfare and later as head of the Sloan-Kettering Institute for Cancer Research. Dr. Rhodes tested the compound and found that it did indeed kill white blood cells and also the bone marrow and lymph cells that produce them. His research confirmed Dr. Alexander's hypothesis, advanced Dr. Gilman's findings and led to the use of mustard compounds to treat cancers of the lymphoid tissues, such as Hodgkin's disease. They are still in use.

At last there was a cancer-killing drug, and the hunt was on for more. In 1947 Dr. Sidney Farber of Boston discovered that the growth of leukemia in mice partially depended on a chemical called folic acid. This led him and his associates to discover another class of chemicals, called folic acid antagonists, which denied the leukemic cells the vital folic acid nutrients. One of the most important of these was aminopterin, a plant extract that proved useful in combating human leukemia. In 1955 the United States Congress approved the first of successive multimillion-dollar appropriations to screen drugs for anticancer activity. A quarter-century later, more than 700,000 natural and synthetic compounds had been studied; from them were winnowed 50 effective anticancer drugs and another 60 that required further trials.

There are four main types of drugs, each interfering with cancer reproduction somewhat differently. One group of the drugs, the alkylating agents, forms chemical bonds of a type called alkyl groups with such important cellular compounds as DNA and RNA *(Chapter 4)*. These bonds short-circuit messages that direct cell division; instead of dividing, the cell dies. Mustargen, cytoxan, alkeran, L-PAM, myleran and BCNU are common alkylating agents.

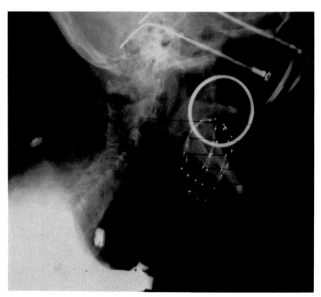

In this side-view X-ray, tiny specks of light are radioactive pellets, set in an oval in and around a tumor at the base of the patient's tongue. The implanted pellets keep cancer-killing radiation close to the tumor, reducing harm to other tissue. A metal ring (set on the skin beneath the patient's glasses) and the black lines on the film are used to check pellet placement.

A second group, called antimetabolites, kills cancers by mimicking substances that are required for cell growth. During the process of multiplication the cell picks up the antimetabolite, which it cannot use, instead of the chemical it needs. Denied an essential ingredient, the cell is unable to divide and it dies. Such drugs as methotrexate, 5-fluorouracil and cytosine arabinoside work this way.

The third type includes antibiotics originally derived from soil fungi, such as daunomycin, adriamycin, bleomycin, actinomycin-D and mutamycin-C. They apparently bind with the DNA molecule and disrupt its myriad functions but, unlike the alkylating agents, do not form alkyl groups.

Anticancer drugs in the fourth group are plant alkaloids derived from periwinkles. They prevent cell division, but unlike the antimetabolites, they do not substitute a dummy compound. Instead, they inhibit the construction of proteins that normally allow the double-stranded DNA to unzip into two single strands, as it must for successful reproduction. Vinblastine and vincristine are the only two plant alkaloids currently sanctioned in the United States but others, including some derived from May apples, are under investigation.

In addition to these drugs, or sometimes in place of them, doctors frequently treat cancer with natural or synthetic hormones. These chemicals, which help regulate growth in animals and plants, can stimulate or retard the development of cancer cells. Some common hormone compounds used include prednisone, diethylstilbestrol (DES) and tamoxifen.

Rarely are any of these drugs used alone. Combinations work better. One drug may kill 99.99 per cent of the body's cancer cells; the remaining percentage, for one reason or another, is resistant to the drug. Because cancer affects trillions of malignant cells, even a killing ratio as high as 99.99 per cent would leave thousands—even millions—of cells untouched. In time, those cells would reproduce, leaving the patient little better off than before drug therapy. But if several drugs are given, the cells missed by one are fairly certain to be killed by the others. In the treatment of Hodgkin's disease, for example, a combination of four drugs known by the acronym MOPP—mustargen, oncovin, prednisone and procarbazine—helped bring the five-year survival rate beyond

50 per cent, even for patients in the most advanced stages.

Not all of a patient's anticancer drugs necessarily are given at the same time. One drug might interfere with another; a combination of several drugs administered together might prove too toxic. What is more, some drugs affect cancer cells only at certain times during the cells' life cycles. Some, such as methotrexate, cytarabine and vinblastine, attack only during cell division; others, such as prednisone, adriamycin and cyclophosphamide, work throughout the cell's life cycle. A pathologist can estimate, by inspecting a few tumor cells under a microscope, when the cells will divide. In this way it is possible to decide which drugs to give and when.

The drugs now in use are purer, less dangerous to the patient and more potent against cancer than the early compounds. They have, wrote Drs. Raymond B. Weiss and Vincent T. DeVita of the NCI, "changed the role of medical treatment of cancer from a 'last-ditch' effort to part of the first-line therapy." Unfortunately, many patients and some doctors still regard chemotherapy as a treatment of last resort. One reason for this view is the drugs' side effects, which are unpleasant and virtually unavoidable.

On his 55th birthday Morris B. Abram, a New York attorney and former President of Brandeis University, visited his doctor for a routine physical. A few days later his doctor asked to see him at once. "That night," recalled Abram, "he sat across a table from me and told me, 'Morris, you have acute myelogenous leukemia,' " a type of blood cancer.

Abram was told that his only chance was chemotherapy. "I had the impression that the treatment was worse than the disease," he said. "My hair would fall out, my heart might be impaired, my liver would probably be affected, my kidneys might suffer. But there was some hope." Abram's prescription was a combination of two drugs, an antibiotic and an antimetabolite. "I was to receive the red peril, daunomycin, that looks like the red clay of my native Georgia, with cytosine arabinoside," he later recalled.

As expected, they did cause trouble. The effects stem from the drugs' shared general characteristic—a tendency to attack rapidly dividing cells. Whatever the drugs do to cancer cells they also do to other rapidly dividing cells—including normal ones vital to good health. In disrupting them, they make the patient vulnerable to the same afflictions associated with radiation treatment—susceptibility to infection, nausea, rashes, hair loss and, particularly in some men, sterility.

Most of these ills are temporary and can be eased by various remedies—marijuana, for example, is increasingly used to curb nausea—but some are serious. The drugs' action on the white blood cells of the body's defense system makes a patient very vulnerable to infections that ordinarily are of little concern. With defenses lowered, a cold transmitted by a visitor can develop into potentially fatal pneumonia; that is an extreme case, but infections often strike patients whose defenses have been lowered by anticancer drugs.

For most chemotherapy patients, sufficient protection against infection is provided by normal caution and antibiotics—Abram's were fed into a vein in his arm. But some people prove so vulnerable that they must be housed temporarily in a totally sanitized environment. This is achieved in a so-called laminar-flow room. The circulation of previously sterilized air is controlled so that it sweeps through the sealed room in smooth streams without eddying—a process called laminar flow; thus all germs are carried away from the patient and out of the room, minimizing the chance of infection. Some patients must live in the room for as long as six weeks.

Although Abram avoided such isolation, his treatments were protracted. Some are completed within a few weeks, but his initial therapy was followed by four years of bimonthly drug sessions. "Each was nauseating, and made me vomit," he wrote. But his cancer was arrested and he survived. In 1979, nearly six years after his diagnosis, Abram gave an address at a cancer society meeting in Atlanta.

Yet despite progress in making drug treatments more effective and less debilitating, not all cases are success stories. None of the standard therapies—drugs, surgery or radiation, alone or in combination—can guarantee results. New treatments are being sought and tested all over the world; more talent and money are invested in cancer research than in the study of any other disease. Because cancer is so feared, and established treatments conjure visions of disastrous side effects and an uncertain outcome, patients and their families desperately seek the newest and most promising therapies. Many turn away from the generally approved treatments—even the experimental ones—and, lured by claims of simple nontoxic cures, opt for unconventional therapy.

Most alternative schemes of treatment are available only at a special clinic, and only from its director. Many of these clinics are in out-of-the-way places or in countries—such as Mexico and some Caribbean nations—where medical practices are not as closely regulated as in the United States or Western Europe. The directors of these clinics range from downright swindlers to scientists and physicians who sincerely believe that they have found uniquely useful remedies. Some may be on the right track. Yet virtually none of the purveyors of unproved cancer treatments, whether deceitful or sincere, allow their case records to be examined by an impartial medical jury; nor do they submit their methods to the rigors of independent, controlled clinical trials. If the methods are tested and fail, the treatment promoter normally responds by criticizing the way the test was run or by claiming to be the victim of a medical conspiracy.

The unproved therapies generally depend on a special diet and a secret drug or ''vitamin.'' Special diets are favored because they are believed to adjust chemical imbalances that supposedly give rise to cancer. (No scientific evidence supports such claims.) The diets can vary from simple raw foods or fasting to complicated regimes that involve unusual concoctions. The Gerson method, for example, named after Dr. Max Gerson of New York City, requires hourly drinks of fresh vegetable juice and calf's liver juice; the potions are followed, four to six times a day, with coffee enemas.

Special medications have an obvious appeal: They make a patient feel his cancer is being attacked. They are usually nontoxic, another attractive quality, and they range from serums drawn from horse blood to extracts taken from apricot pits. The latter—marketed as laetrile or vitamin B-17—is the most famous of the unproved anticancer drugs. It is, however, toxic and in certain doses, administered orally, it has caused death by poisoning.

Laetrile was first promoted as an anticancer drug in the 1950s by Dr. Ernest T. Krebs Sr. of San Francisco. Until his death in 1970, at the age of 93, Dr. Krebs was the leader of a large laetrile cult. He personally treated thousands of patients, and his disciples treated thousands more. By 1980 more than 50,000 patients a year were receiving the drug—some of it smuggled into areas where its use is illegal.

Many patients using laetrile have volunteered stirring testimonials to its effectiveness. Yet in nearly all cases, medical records, treatment plans, tests and other essentials of a documented case history are absent. Some patients had received orthodox treatments first, or along with laetrile.

Meanwhile, convincing indictments of laetrile have come from one carefully controlled study after another. Five times between 1957 and 1975, NCI tested laetrile to see whether it inhibited tumor spread or growth in laboratory animals. Five times it failed. And finally it failed an elaborate trial on 156 cancer patients by four major institutions: the Mayo Clinic, the Memorial Sloan-Kettering Cancer Center, the University of California at Los Angeles and the University of Arizona. Said Dr. Charles G. Moertel of the Mayo Clinic, ''Laetrile has been tested. It is not effective.''

The inability of treatments such as laetrile to withstand rigorous scrutiny indicates the hazard of relying on them. They delay therapy that is known to help—and may delay it so long it becomes futile.

Far-out ideas that may work

To warn against the presently unproved cancer treatments, however, is not to say that all will be so forever. Today's accepted therapies were also, at one time or another, unproved. By now all have passed carefully controlled trials, publicly documented and confirmed repeatedly by separate, independent investigations. Many still-unproved treatments are in this research stage. Two of the most promising are hyperthermia, heating tumors to inhibit their growth, and immunotherapy, stimulating the body's natural defenses to destroy or neutralize malignant cells.

The idea that elevated body temperature might inhibit tumor growth has been around since the 1860s. Dr. Leon C. Parks of the University of Mississippi confirmed this effect in 1980. He devised a procedure in which a patient's blood is

The cancer subculture: unorthodox treatments

Each year, thousands of desperate cancer patients forsake their own physicians and troop to practitioners of unproved and unconventional therapies. It is easy to understand why. Many of the patients have undergone standard treatments in vain and are lured by the promise of a cure that does not mutilate, nauseate or burn. Clinics offering such therapies exist in many countries, but most are in Mexico (where the pictures on the following pages were taken), the United States, West Germany, the Philippines and the Bahamas. They range from expensive, well-equipped hospitals to picturesque "health resorts" and cut-rate dispensaries.

Some of their therapies are unconventional because their efficacy—or lack of it—is not yet established unequivocally. Other treatments are known to have some value yet may be limited. But many are gimmicks—questionable drugs, air "ionizers" and special-posture beds. One clinic in Mexico offers the gamut: Computers analyze a patient's condition, then doctors tailor a program that usually involves a health-food diet and doses of laetrile, a controversial drug derived from apricot pits.

Purveyors of unorthodox cancer therapies claim stunning triumphs; independent studies do not back them up. Still, stories of miracles abound. A visitor to a Mexican cancer clinic offered one explanation—the pilgrimage effect. "You've come all the way to a strange place," he said, "and you're more likely to experience a miracle here than in Elm City General Hospital back home."

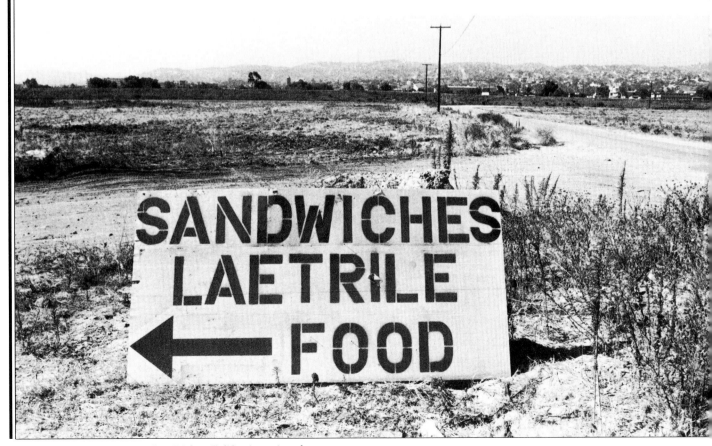

A sign on a dusty road near San Ysidro, California, points the way to the Mexican border, one mile south, where the drug laetrile can be purchased legally. Laetrile repeatedly has been found ineffective in fighting cancer and is banned in 29 states. But some 50,000 United States citizens who have cancer rely on it.

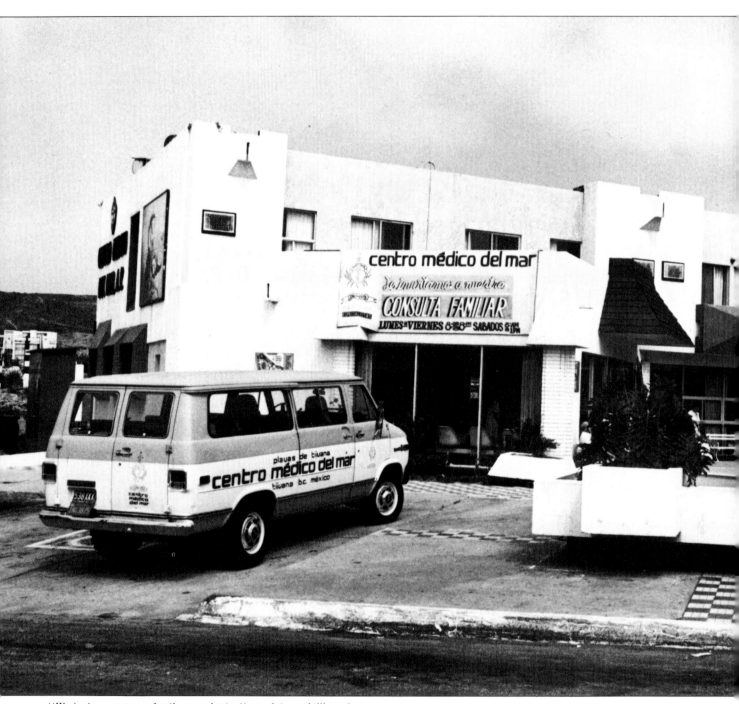

"We invite you to our family consultation" proclaims a billboard over the entrance to the posh Del Mar Medical Center in Tijuana, Mexico. The Clinic specializes in a "holistic" approach to cancer care, offering conventional and unconventional drugs—including laetrile—and psychological therapies that aim to mobilize the mind to fight the disease.

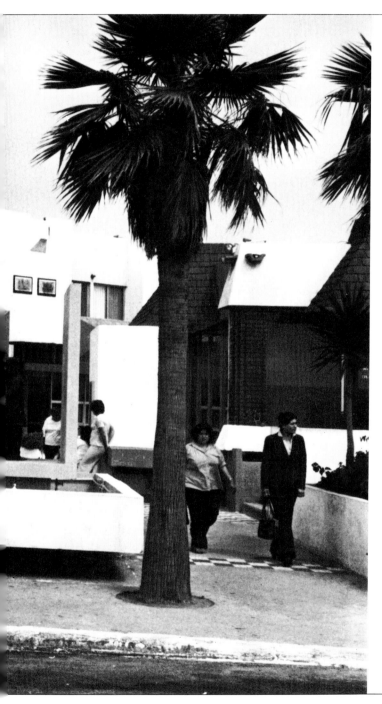

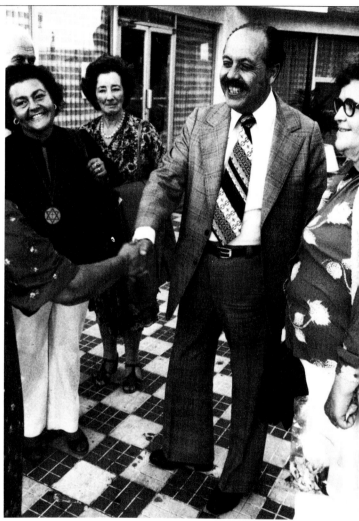

Dr. Ernesto Contreras, founder and proprietor of the Del Mar Medical Center, welcomes visitors and prospective patients to his clinic. Since the mid-1960s, when Dr. Contreras began to dispense laetrile from an office in his home, he has treated more than 35,000 cancer patients from the United States and has built a multimillion-dollar medical empire.

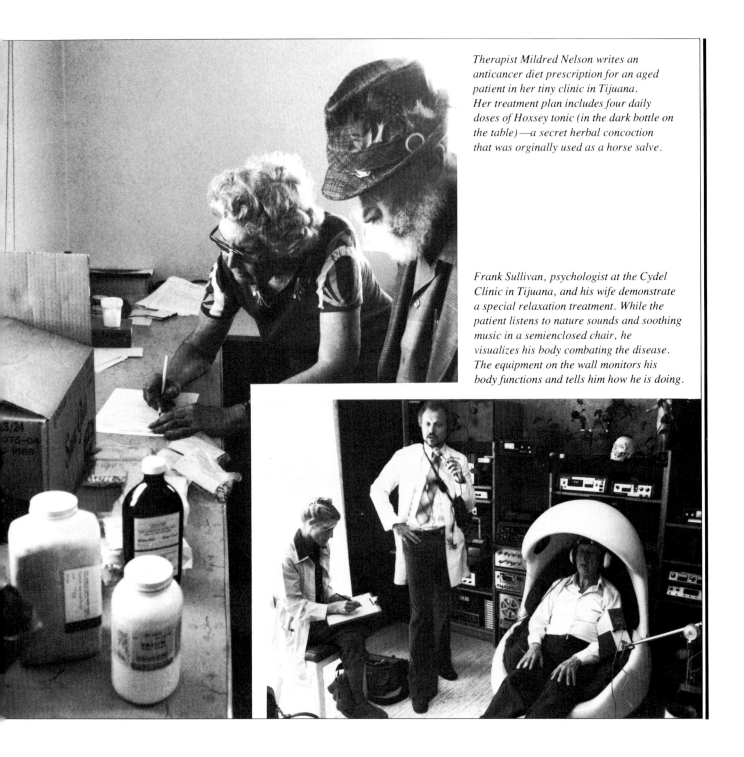

Therapist Mildred Nelson writes an anticancer diet prescription for an aged patient in her tiny clinic in Tijuana. Her treatment plan includes four daily doses of Hoxsey tonic (in the dark bottle on the table)—a secret herbal concoction that was orginally used as a horse salve.

Frank Sullivan, psychologist at the Cydel Clinic in Tijuana, and his wife demonstrate a special relaxation treatment. While the patient listens to nature sounds and soothing music in a semienclosed chair, he visualizes his body combating the disease. The equipment on the wall monitors his body functions and tells him how he is doing.

withdrawn from his body through a tube and then passed through a heating coil. Warmed to 106.7° F.—8.1 degrees above normal—the blood is then returned to the patient, who meanwhile receives low doses of drugs and, in some cases, radiation. The procedure takes from four to eight hours.

The results obtained by Dr. Parks were encouraging, if tentative. Of 104 patients in one test group—"all with far-advanced malignancies," he said—tumors disappeared in 15 and shrank 50 per cent or more in 12 others. Apparently, heat made the tumors more sensitive to radiation and drugs.

Even greater hope is attached to schemes for arousing the body's natural defenses. Such immunotherapy stimulates the immune system, the very complex of disease-fighting mechanisms that is harmed by radiation and anticancer drugs, to operate more efficiently and rid the body of cancer cells. The therapy depends on the fact that cancer cells are not normal constituents of the body. They are in effect foreign. Like all foreign invaders of the body, they should be vulnerable to attack—if the immune system is active enough. In one experimental technique tested successfully on laboratory animals, doctors remove a cluster of tumor cells. The cells are killed and then treated with chemicals or radiation to make them appear more foreign to the body. The treated cells are then reimplanted, on the theory that they will provoke an immune response to other tumor cells in the body.

Better results with human subjects have been achieved with a technique called nonspecific immunotherapy, which was devised originally to combat tuberculosis. Long ago, medical scientists noted that patients who had recovered from one kind of infection became more resistant to other infections. The immunity developed by the first illness somehow kept the system mobilized so that it could fight off different illnesses. This fact was exploited in 1922 by Leon Calmette and Camille Guérin of France to develop the tuberculosis vaccine named for them, Bacillus-Calmette-Guérin, or BCG. It has been widely employed in antituberculosis campaigns in Europe, although it is little used in the United States. BCG, it turns out, also seems to work against cancer when the drug is combined with conventional therapy.

Although some trials of BCG have been disappointing—a British study of 92 lung-cancer patients from Nottingham and Sheffield noted insignificant improvement from use of the vaccine—a number of other investigations in the United States and France found that it improved survival from some kinds of cancers. In one experiment at the Albany Medical College and affiliated hospitals, only two of 26 early-stage lung-cancer patients treated with BCG plus other therapies experienced recurring cancer within three to four years; nine of 32 who did not receive BCG had a relapse.

For another, much-touted immune-system stimulant—interferon—the reviews are similarly mixed. In one landmark trial, Dr. Hans Strander of Karolinska Hospital in Stockholm treated some 35 bone-cancer patients with interferon. A similarly sized group did not receive the drug. Of the 35 treated with interferon, almost two thirds showed no sign of cancer spread 30 months after diagnosis. Of those who did not receive the drug, nearly 70 per cent did show signs of cancer spread. On the other hand, a study at the Memorial Sloan-Kettering Cancer Center was less successful. Of 15 lung-cancer patients treated with interferon and evaluated, eight showed no change, and seven grew worse.

"Immunotherapy is still in its infancy," said the French cancer specialist Dr. Lucien Israël, "yet those who have had long enough experience with the various procedures of immunotherapy are convinced that something is going on, and that we may not be far from some very exciting results."

Exciting results have already been seen in the other forms of cancer treatments. Thanks to advances in the use of surgery, radiation and drugs, millions of people who a few years ago would have died now live out their normal lives. And the pace of advance accelerates. The optimism of Dr. Israël applies to all kinds of cancer therapy. He spoke for researchers and practicing physicians the world over when he said: "I am physically tired from almost monthly trips to the United States or elsewhere, where in two days we communicate to one another our observations on the latest improvements that have been thought up in this daily battle. But there is hardly a trip from which I don't return with some small, encouraging innovation, some slight advance or some project based on an encouraging observation."   ✳

CHAPTER 6

Coping with cancer

A new way to speak
After breast surgery, a normal life and appearance
Countering the side effects of drugs and rays
How patients help patients
When treatment fails

For a cancer patient, the process of dealing successfully with the disease begins at the moment of diagnosis. When 13-year-old John Filbeck learned he had a cancer near his spine, his first question was, "Will I die?" Told that he probably would not, he asked, "Can I play football again?" (John did not die; he did play football again.) When 16-year-old Jeanna Kelly was told that she had bone cancer and that the treatment for it would cause her to lose her wavy hair, she wept and yelled and threw things in a healthy display of anger.

The responses of these teenagers were direct and immediate. Adults are likely to have delayed, mixed reactions to a diagnosis of cancer in themselves or a family member—reactions as diverse as the modes and scopes of treatment and rehabilitation. Most patients are confronted with the trauma of surgery—and often the aftermath of surgery, when artificial devices take the place of excised organs. Others live for weeks or months with the side effects of therapeutic radiation or anticancer drugs. After treatment there are individual problems of returning to school or a job, and for some, the realization that the disease has advanced to a stage where death is inescapable.

But for all there is a moment of shock and confusion when a doctor announces the diagnosis. "Your emotions run the gamut from disbelief to fear to feelings of great loss," reported Rose Bird, Chief Justice of California, a breast cancer victim. "Disbelief, because cancer is always something that happens to the next person, not to you. Fear, because everyone living in this society has been conditioned to believe that

a diagnosis of cancer is equivalent to a death warrant."

How adults cope with the news depends in part on how they are used to coping with other crises of life. Justice Bird had never had a serious illness, and her first reaction was a common one: denial. She refused to learn anything about her disease, and as soon as her surgery and recuperation were over she plunged back into her demanding schedule. For a time, she confessed, she became a workaholic as a way of running away from her fear of a recurrence. Eventually, when a recurrence did take place, Justice Bird faced the fact of her cancer, and her response shifted from denial to sober concern. "I began to read as much of the literature as I could," she said. "I felt I needed to know as much as the doctors did."

Rose Bird's decision to study cancer and her own case helped her because, quite simply, the facts are seldom as frightening as the fears. The basic fact, of course, is that today most cancers are curable. Beyond this, most patients deal better with fears and anxieties when they know exactly what is wrong and what can be done. Such facts are increasingly easy to find out—but not everywhere. In some countries, cancer is hushed up. In France, for example, according to Catherine Adonis, a French nurse specializing in cancer care, "the vast majority of our patients remain unaware, or apparently unaware, of their diagnosis. Curious though it may seem, most patients never even ask to be told the truth. This attitude is proof enough that they have their suspicions but it also reflects their desire to remain in doubt, to entertain

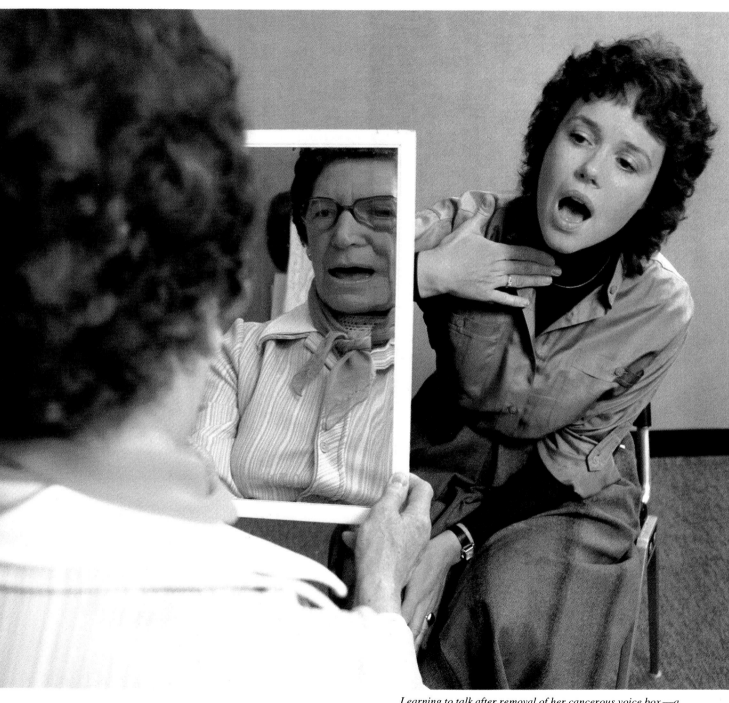

Learning to talk after removal of her cancerous voice box—a laryngectomy, which closes the windpipe—a patient positions her tongue with the help of a speech therapist. The tongue forces air into the esophagus, or gullet. Throat contractions force the air back to the mouth, making a sound. A collar protects a throat opening that enables the patient to breathe air into her lungs.

the delusion that they may have some other disease.''

This response is discouraged elsewhere; in most countries, the medical profession increasingly believes that facing the facts is an important part of the cure. ''When the truth is withheld, formidable problems arise,'' said the English medical journal *The Lancet*. ''Patients usually have some notion of what is wrong with them before they see a doctor and may imagine the diagnosis to be worse than it actually is, but the necessary reassurance is impossible if the diagnosis is not mentioned.''

The matter is slightly different when children are the patients, especially when the child is quite young and the cancer is difficult to cure. According to clinical psychologist Maria H. Nagy, of the Columbia Presbyterian Medical Center in New York City, children under the age of nine do not have a realistic notion of the meaning of death. Preschool children fear separation from their families but do not expect to die ''for good''; children between the ages of six and nine fear mutilation but do not generally recognize death as a universal fate—although they may be terrified by the thought of their own death.

From this knowledge of children's perception of death, some authorities have arrived at guidelines for informing young patients about their diagnosis. These experts suggest that a toddler be told only that he is sick and needs to cooperate in his treatments in order to get better. The serious nature of the illness can be conveyed to an older child, but he must be constantly reassured that his disease is treatable—many young people, misled by fragments of information they have picked up, believe everyone who contracts cancer will die.

Among adults, there are probably as many ways of finding strength to deal with the emotional shock of cancer as there are people. Some find it in religion, others in the support of families and friends. When columnist Stewart Alsop was first hospitalized for tests, his wife Tish went with him, and when it became apparent that he had cancer, he wrote, ''I was afraid and reached out for her hand, which felt warm and comforting and very much alive.'' On Alsop's first night in the hospital his wife stayed on a cot by his bed. ''Twice I woke up, despite the sleeping pill I had taken, and was afraid and reached for Tish's hand. Both times she was awake.''

Confidence in doctors and nurses helps, too. When the 43-year-old California writer Ellen Abbott discovered that she had ovarian cancer, she decided that she was not going to worry about the details of her treatment. ''That's their problem,'' she told herself. ''I have enough to do handling my family and friends and everybody else, doing all the things I want to do. Naturally, I tell them my symptoms and cooperate with them. I do everything they tell me, but basically all of the therapy is up to them; I don't have to worry about it.''

For many the best weapon in the battle is a simple determination to go on living—and what is more, to live a normal life. When 27-year-old university teacher Nick Tanis was told he had cancer his immediate response, as he later recalled it, was: '' 'Dammit, I'm going to live!' Whatever happened, I wasn't going to give in.'' He did not—and missed only two classes during his years of treatment. Equally often, a resolve to live as normally as possible is calm and deliberate. Mort Segal, a hard-working, successful California lawyer who was stricken with a rare cancer at the age of 40, continued to carry on his profession at almost his usual pace throughout the course of his illness. ''If you feel good about yourself, if you are doing what you want to do, you don't change your life just because you're sick,'' he said.

The truth is that most people, one way or another, find inner strength to confront the difficulties of a serious illness with determination and even cheerfulness. ''There is a general feeling among the public and physicians that all cancer patients are depressed,'' said Dr. Jimmie Holland, Chief of Psychiatric Service at Memorial Sloan-Kettering Cancer Center in New York. This, she said, ''is a myth,'' adding, ''True depression, which occurs in only a small percentage of cancer patients, should be vigorously treated by psychiatric intervention, including psychotherapy and, often, antidepressant medication.''

A new way to speak

If any therapy arouses justifiable anxiety and depression, it is an operation to remove a cancerous organ or tissue. Yet surgery offers the best cure for most tumors, and although the aftereffects cannot be eliminated, they can be compensated for. An artificial body part, or prosthesis (from the Greek word for "an addition"), takes the place of an organ or limb lost to the disease. Plastic surgery restores the appearance of surgically damaged areas. Specialized therapies and techniques make up for the loss of such functions as speech.

Some of these aids are conventional devices—the removal of an arm or leg because of bone cancer is not different from the same loss in an automobile accident and is compensated for with an artificial arm or leg. Three areas of the body, however, are frequent sites of cancer operations that require special types of postsurgery treatment. One such area is the head and neck, affected by several kinds of surgery. Another is the breast, all or part of which may be removed. A third is the lower intestine and rectum, partly excised during a colostomy.

About a third of all head and neck cancer patients require a prosthesis to restore function, improve appearance or both. The most common, an obturator, is a plastic plug that seals off a hole or cavity left by surgery, usually in the soft palate or upper jaw. When the obturator is set in place a few days after surgery, the patient regains the ability to take food by mouth and to speak.

One of the most common head and neck cancers strikes the larynx, or vocal cords. It can be cured in almost 60 per cent of the cases. The common treatment is surgery, which removes the larynx entirely and deprives the patient of the normal mechanism for speech. Electronic voice boxes have been devised, but most often the patient learns to talk without any larynx, using esophageal speech. Classroom lessons over a period that may last three months teach him to swallow air, then release it slowly through the esophagus while articulating words with the tongue, teeth and lips. Three out of five patients master the new skills.

The successes of this therapy can be astounding. When actor William Gargan lost his voice after a laryngectomy, he also lost his career, and he might have retreated into a lonely, silent life. What made the difference was a speech-therapy program. Before long Gargan was not only enjoying a normal social life but making speeches all over the United States in aid of other cancer victims. Another throat cancer patient, schoolteacher Anne Gibson Lanpher, learned esophageal speech in record time. Four months after her larynx was removed she was traveling in France and talking so normally that few of her hearers thought she had anything worse than a sore throat. At the end of six months she was back at her job—teaching her students to enunciate French.

Although the technique of esophageal speech is simple in principle, it can be acquired only after long practice. If the patient becomes frustrated, or if his family and friends are not sufficiently understanding, he may give up attempting esophageal speech and resort to the simpler but psychologically isolating expedient of writing down his thoughts. Loss of voice all too often leads to social withdrawal.

A greater danger of withdrawal arises when head surgery drastically alters appearance. The operation may have been a surgical success but, said Dr. Vincent R. Hentz of the Stanford University School of Medicine, "a cure under these circumstances is meaningless." The jaw or face must be restored to a natural appearance by plastic surgery; several reconstruction operations may be needed.

After breast surgery, a normal life and appearance

Change in physical appearance may also result from surgery for breast cancer, particularly if such a mastectomy removes large amounts of tissue, as is often the case. This change in appearance is frequently blamed for psychological trauma, but the trauma has apparently been exaggerated. A study at Massachusetts General Hospital showed that, six months after surgery, four out of five of the breast cancer patients were no more depressed, withdrawn or lacking in self-esteem than a random sampling of nonpatients. What is more, the 20 per cent who did show signs of depression apparently had had psychological problems before their surgery—problems that were unrelated to cancer.

Whatever the psychological effect of a mastectomy, it need not stem from fears about appearance. For the woman who has had a breast removed, department stores, surgical-supply houses and specialized boutiques provide a special brassiere. One cup is of the usual kind; the other has a pocket for a fluid-filled prosthesis designed to match both the shape and the weight of the intact breast (the weight must be the same on both sides of the chest to prevent back strain). Mastectomy boutiques also carry swimsuits and nightgowns with built-in foam-rubber cups. The variety of these devices is endless. They can, for example, be adapted for a woman who has had both breasts removed. And even if a radical, or deep, mastectomy has been performed on one side of the chest and a simple, or shallow, one on the other, the differences between the two can be compensated for in the size of the inserts and the construction of the garment.

Women who choose to go beyond such prostheses to plastic surgery may undergo a second and sometimes a third operation to have their breasts reconstructed. This surgery can begin as early as three months after a mastectomy. A silicone-filled envelope is implanted under the skin to form a breast mound. Later, the surgeon may reconstruct a nipple by grafting skin from a part of the body with a similar color and texture, such as the nipple of the other breast—in some cases the nipple from the removed breast can be saved and "banked" for use in the reconstruction. Until recently, only one out of a hundred mastectomy patients had breast reconstructions, but the number has been rapidly rising as techniques improve; in the United States, for example, approximately 15,000 women have had breasts rebuilt.

The psychological effect of such reconstruction can turn a

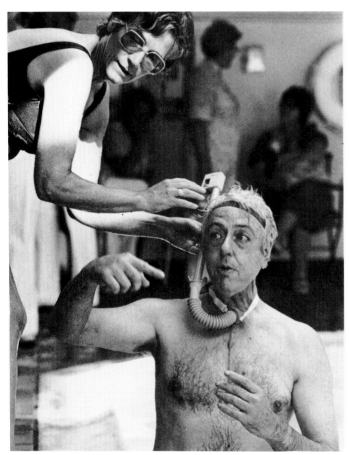

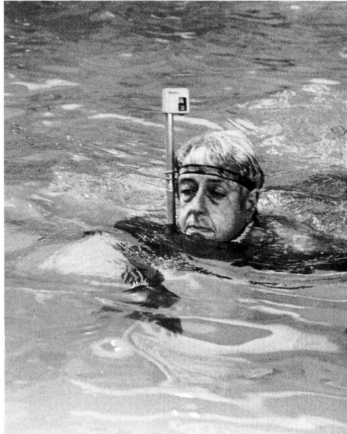

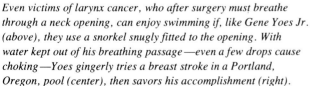

Even victims of larynx cancer, who after surgery must breathe through a neck opening, can enjoy swimming if, like Gene Yoes Jr. (above), they use a snorkel snugly fitted to the opening. With water kept out of his breathing passage—even a few drops cause choking—Yoes gingerly tries a breast stroke in a Portland, Oregon, pool (center), then savors his accomplishment (right).

woman's life around. After a mastectomy, Dallas art dealer Susan Morgan spent two years, she said, ''getting undressed in a closet.'' But after one look at her reconstructed breast, she ''couldn't stop grinning.'' The reconstruction, she concluded, ''changed my life in a more positive way than being sick changed it in a negative way.''

Prostheses and plastic surgery may be options after a mastectomy, but special therapies and precautions often are a necessity. In radical and modified-radical operations, lymph nodes or muscles are removed as well as the breast itself, and their functions must be protected or restored. Many women follow systematic programs of exercise to strengthen muscles and reestablish normal shoulder movement. Without such exercises, the shoulder near the removed lymph nodes may become stiff and painful.

Unlike breast cancer patients, those who have had part of their intestines removed in colostomies need prostheses for function rather than for appearance. After the cancerous part of the intestine is cut away, the surgeon generally makes an opening in the skin called a stoma, through which body wastes can be released. A replaceable plastic pouch fitted tightly into the stoma receives the wastes. The pouch must be cleaned every time it is used; the stoma must be thoroughly washed off and flushed of wastes, a process called irrigation. These procedures are time-consuming. Irrigating the stoma can take an hour or more. Some patients irrigate every two or

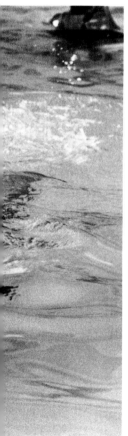
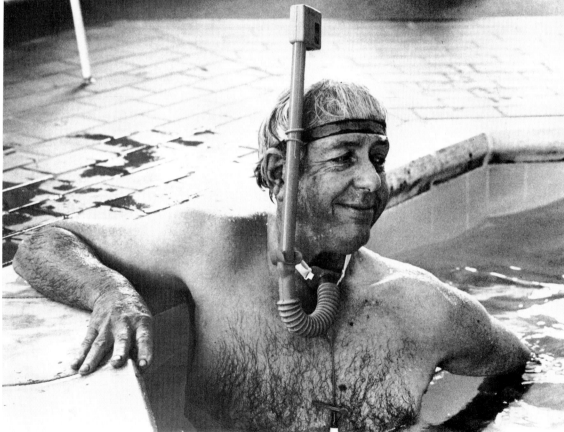

three days, others must irrigate daily. Whatever the schedule, the patient must stick to it, so that the digestive system functions with regularity.

Most patients quickly adapt to the routine. When Letitia Baldrige, head of her own public relations firm in New York City, woke up from an operation for cancer of the colon and learned that she was a member of what she called "the plastic bag set," she simply resolved to accept it. "To me, the plastic bag seemed a small price for survival." To help her learn the use of the new appliance and how to integrate it into her daily life, she and other members of "the set" had the help of trained specialists, whose work begins even before the operation.

Working with the surgeon, one specialist helps plan the location of the stoma so that it will interfere with everyday activities as little as possible and be easy for the patient to take care of. After the operation nurses check every day to see that the new appliance is functioning properly, to teach the patient how to use it, and—equally important—to reassure him about its effect on his daily life (no, it need not smell; no, it will not show; yes, he can have a full sexual life). When a patient goes home a visiting nurse may see him regularly until he learns to manage on his own.

Countering the side effects of drugs and rays

Adapting to life after treatment is not a problem for patients in chemotherapy and radiotherapy. Their shocks of reality come during treatment, not afterward. These techniques, or combinations of them, are responsible for the most startling advances in modern cancer treatment, but they can be grueling. The powerful drugs and rays not only destroy tumor cells and prevent new ones from forming, but also destroy some normal cells and adversely affect other healthy, rapidly growing cells in the bone marrow, the intestinal tract, the reproductive organs and the hair follicles. Most of these side effects can be ameliorated by simple efforts of the patient or by drugs, some new, some old.

Cancer-killing chemicals in particular are so potent that most patients take a routine blood test before every session; if previous sessions have destroyed too many blood cells, creating a threat of anemia, the treatment may be postponed. But even under the best conditions the chemicals are likely to destroy large numbers of platelets, the parts of red blood cells that cause blood to clot, and many patients are plagued by bleeding. Patients must learn to take small precautions that always help but are sometimes overlooked. To prevent nosebleed, they must avoid forceful blowing; they must brush their teeth with toothbrushes having the softest bristles and shave with electric razors—and of course exercise special care when using knives.

Perhaps the most distressing side effect of chemotherapy is nausea and vomiting. Some patients report only brief spells of queasiness, but most experience severe nausea. Obviously, the latter group is in need of an effective antiemetic. A number are effective, including trimethobenzamide, promethazine and prochlorperazine. Unfortunately, however, the one that is most useful is also the most controversial and difficult to obtain. It is tetrahydrocannabinol, or THC, the active ingredient in marijuana.

THC not only counteracts nausea but is a good sedative, sometimes masks pain and stimulates the appetite (loss of appetite is a frequent side effect of chemotherapy, and anything that makes eating appealing can be a blessing). It also has side effects of its own. Older patients, particularly, dislike the feeling of being high and of losing some measure of muscular control. And in the United States neither refined THC nor crude marijuana is available by prescription, although the National Cancer Institute began in 1980 to distribute THC capsules to certain research physicians conducting clinical tests on cancer patients. Nevertheless, some doctors encourage law-abiding patients to smoke illegal marijuana on the sly before a chemotherapy session.

Outside the United States, doctors have much greater freedom in prescribing drugs, and some order marijuana for their cancer patients. In England, the narcotic heroin is used to relieve the pain of cancer, and many Americans have pressed for similar use of heroin in the United States. However, several studies have demonstrated that, although heroin is one of the strongest and most easily assimilated of the powerful painkillers, other drugs such as morphine can serve as well if properly administered. The director of one investigation, Dr. Raymond Houde of Memorial Sloan-Kettering Cancer Institute, concluded that there is "no indication that heroin has any unique advantages over morphine."

Less serious than nausea as an aftereffect of chemotherapy is baldness—the chemicals used in chemotherapy attack the hair follicles. Tightly tied tourniquets or turbans filled with ice cubes can sometimes reduce the flow of chemical-laden blood to the scalp during treatments; in any case hair growth starts again three to four weeks after the treatment ends. In the meantime the patient may use a simple prosthesis—a wig. Sixteen-year-old Jeanna Kelly had a different, but effective, idea. "Wigs are not normal," she declared, and wore bright scarves and floppy hats instead. "If you can't have hair," she said, "have style." Young John Filbeck flaunted his baldness with boldness, as though it were a new fad in hairdos.

Many side effects of radiation therapy, including hair loss and nausea, are similar to those of chemotherapy; in addition, irradiated patients almost always suffer from fatigue and from patches of sensitive skin that may be dry, itchy and darkened. But many of the effects of radiation arise only in localized areas where the beams are tightly focused: Hair loss occurs mainly when the scalp, chest or pubic area is irradiated; nausea, when the stomach is treated; damaged skin, in the area struck by the beam. Often, radiation patients have one special psychological problem: an understandable fear of the powerful beams that are trained upon them. Some of their worst fears are without foundation. Radiation does not make the patient radioactive. It does not hurt at all—and the treatment generally lasts only about two minutes.

Because of the side effects of chemotherapy and radiation, patients are tempted to miss sessions. That temptation may be the most dangerous side effe t of all. As Dr. Charlotte Jacobs, Director of the Oncology Day Care Center at Stanford University Medical Center, expressed it: "The curable cancers are curable only if the patient comes regularly for treatment."

Inventive scheduling can help. Mara Flaherty, a 33-year-old writer afflicted with bone cancer, was determined to keep up with her chemotherapy and radiation treatments—and equally determined to prevent them from disrupting her life. She set her sessions for late Friday every week. That way she could put in a normal work week, recuperate all day Saturday and see friends on Sunday. When another young woman found that her radiation therapy at Massachusetts General

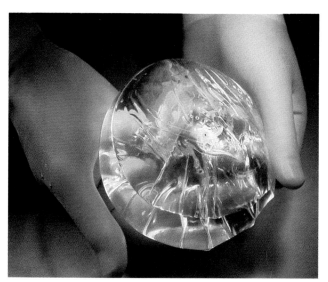

A permanent implant that restores breast shape after a mastectomy, shown here fully assembled, consists of a flexible silicone shell containing a thick silicone fluid. The implant is inserted through an incision in chest muscles.

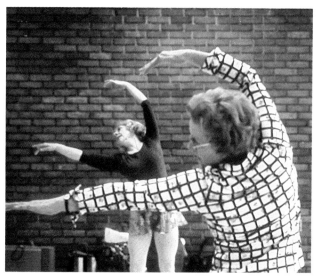

Following an instructor's lead, a woman recovering from breast surgery (foreground) performs a stretching exercise at the Princeton, New Jersey, YWCA. Such exercises, which restore strength to arm and chest muscles weakened by the surgery, are part of a program that also aids emotional recovery by encouraging women to share experiences and exchange advice.

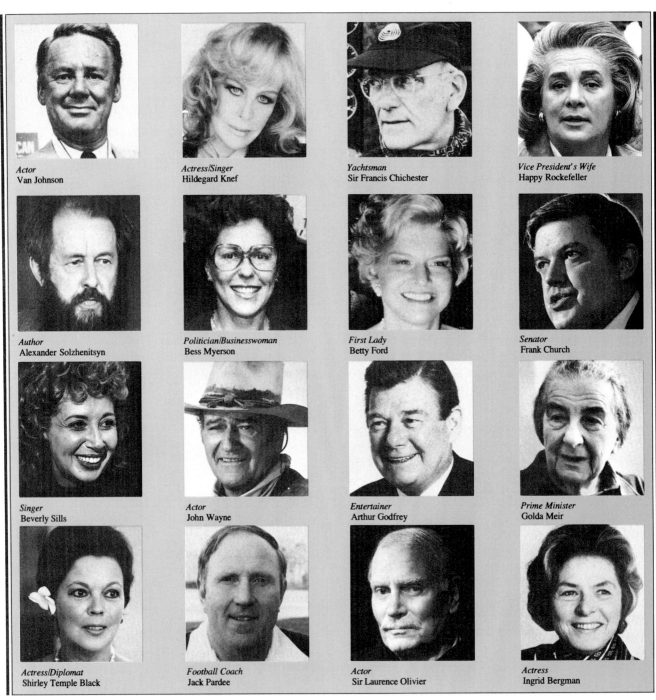

Actor
Van Johnson

Actress/Singer
Hildegard Knef

Yachtsman
Sir Francis Chichester

Vice President's Wife
Happy Rockefeller

Author
Alexander Solzhenitsyn

Politician/Businesswoman
Bess Myerson

First Lady
Betty Ford

Senator
Frank Church

Singer
Beverly Sills

Actor
John Wayne

Entertainer
Arthur Godfrey

Prime Minister
Golda Meir

Actress/Diplomat
Shirley Temple Black

Football Coach
Jack Pardee

Actor
Sir Laurence Olivier

Actress
Ingrid Bergman

The lives of these 16 famous men and women attest to the
success of modern cancer treatment. All of them continued to be
active and productive for at least seven years after diagnosis.

Hospital made it impossible for her to keep her food down, she rearranged her day. She rose at four in the morning for breakfast and ate lunch at eight—giving her plenty of time to digest her food before an afternoon treatment. Mara Flaherty spoke for both of the women and for thousands of other patients when she remarked: "We're all a lot tougher than we think. We don't have to fall apart, and we don't need continual assistance."

How patients help patients

The key word in Mara's remark may be "continual." Few cancer patients need help continually; almost all need it from time to time. The long period after treatment—a period of adjustment to a new life while simultaneously the threads of the old one are picked up—calls for concerned and expert aid. Though warm, supportive attitudes in family and friends help the cancer victim in his efforts to cope, there often comes a moment when an expatient feels isolated and alone, especially when treatment results in a crippling or disfiguring loss. Friends and family members, not having experienced these problems themselves, can offer but limited comfort. At such moments, contact with other cancer patients who have succeeded in returning to normal life can be invaluable.

Such contacts are now a standard part of posttreatment therapy. They are arranged largely by volunteer organizations. Reach to Recovery, for example, deals with the problems of women who have undergone breast surgery. The United Ostomy Association and informal ostomy clubs in many countries give psychological support and recommend services and equipment to colostomy patients. The Candlelighters, an organization of parents whose children suffer from cancer, advises on ways to maintain a normal home life. The International Association of Laryngectomees assists its members, who have just learned to speak in an unaccustomed manner, in their relationships with employers. And all these organizations help patients adhere to life-enhancing regimens—to stop smoking, to practice exercises that restore normal movement, to learn to use prostheses.

The work of these groups sometimes begins before a patient leaves the hospital. "I had never heard of Reach to Recovery before," said Thelma Palmerio, a New Yorker who had a mastectomy at the age of 43, "but my doctor and the nurse on duty told me someone would be coming. The night before I was released, this perky blonde came in—her name was Nadine. She was in her mid-thirties and I remember that she wore a tight sweater." Nadine had also had a mastectomy, and the obviousness of that sweater made Thelma Palmerio laugh. "But it worked!" she said. "I had been feeling like my life was over. Coming out of anesthesia, my first thoughts were that I could never get medical insurance again and that I could never change jobs. The next thought was that no man would ever look at me again. But Nadine was about to get married in a month."

Thelma Palmerio's own good experience led her to become a volunteer herself. "I've never gotten as much satisfaction out of anything in my life," she said. "You get instant feedback, instant reaction. I've gone in feeling depressed myself and come out feeling invigorated. It's a shot in the arm."

While mutual-help organizations do much to provide a bridge back to normal life, returning to work can itself be the best therapy for a cancer patient. According to Bonnie Denmark Friedman, a medical social worker, "People who resume work show fewer signs of low self-esteem, poor morale, anxiety and depression, and seem to feel less threatened by cancer than do their nonworking counterparts." Some cancer patients, however, report that the disease has made work difficult to find. It is not that they cannot meet the demands of a job; in many cases they have recovered their full strength and capacities. The problem is in the attitude of some employers who regard cancer with a sort of superstitious dread, as though the disease were contagious, or who think that the recovered patient is a doomed person, one whose days are numbered.

Such prejudice is baseless, as shown in a study by the Metropolitan Life Insurance Company. Between 1957 and 1971, the company hired 74 people who had suffered from cancer; 43 were hired less than five years after treatment. At the end of the period, 41 of the employees were still working, two were disabled and the remaining 31 had left their jobs

Where the specialty is tender loving care

Tucked into a London suburb, St. Christopher's Hospice does not look like a place that is about dying. It has a greenhouse and gardens, sun porches, floor-to-ceiling windows. Yet its 62 tenants—nearly all of them cancer victims—are there to live out their last weeks. Founded in 1967, St. Christopher's is a pioneer of hospice care, an expanding medical specialty devoted to patients who cannot be cured. Fifty such programs exist in the United Kingdom; more than 200 have sprung up in the United States.

Hospices do what hospitals seldom can. A dying person can feel a failure in an institution whose staff is oriented to making people well. Hospice doctors, nurses and volunteers have a different mission: They comfort the patients, lavish attention and affection on each one and help each to find meaning in life and death.

The patients have a say in their hospice treatment. Pain-killing drugs are available as needed, not according to the rigid schedule of a hospital. Patients' beds are surrounded with personal furnishings and souvenirs; family and friends are always welcome. And the staff tries never to be too busy to rub a back or share a patient's anger and fears. "We extend the quality of life," said a hospice official, "when we can't extend the quantity."

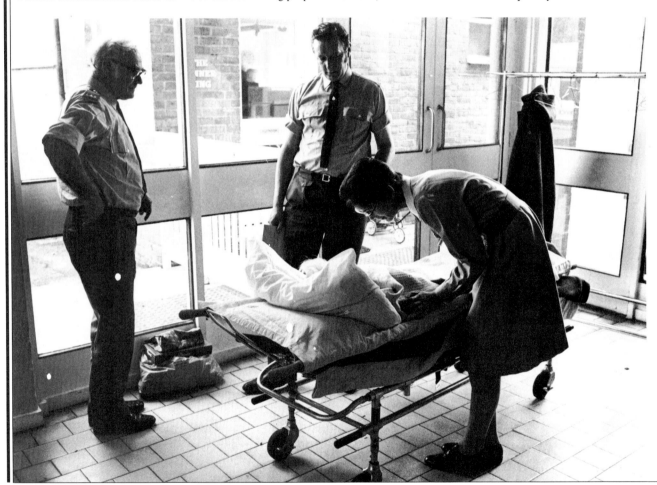

A warm, intimate welcome from Helen Willans, nursing director of St. Christopher's Hospice, expresses the hospice's family atmosphere as she greets a patient just brought in by ambulance drivers. "She does that for everyone," said a patient. "I looked at her face and could see that she was glad to have me."

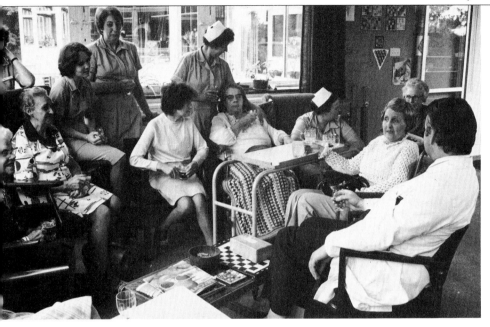

*Patients and staff members gather in
an activities room for their weekly cocktail
hour. Loneliness is seldom a problem at
St. Christopher's. The patients get together
for poetry workshops and painting classes,
and they play with staff members' children,
who have a nursery on the grounds.*

*The Hospice's Anglican chaplain makes his
Sunday rounds to offer communion. A
weekly Roman Catholic Mass is celebrated
as well at St. Christopher's, which
is a nonsectarian institution not directly
affiliated with any church.*

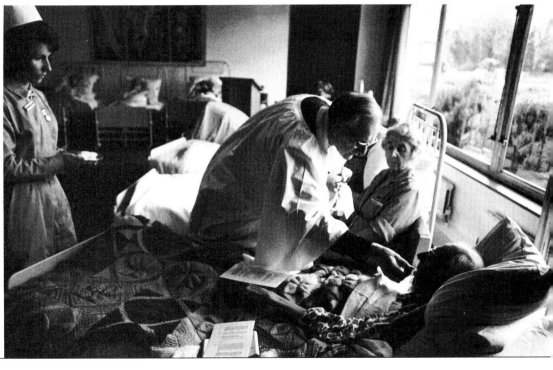

Hospice in the home

Following the lead of St. Christopher's in London, many hospitals have created hospice teams of specially trained doctors and nurses to treat terminally ill patients. Most common in the United States, however, are hospices that treat patients at home, enabling them to finish life with a measure of independence in the place that means the most to them.

Most home-care hospices are nonprofit organizations established by local nurses, physicians and clergy, who enlist volunteers to raise funds and assist patients with household chores and transportation. Among the advantages of such home-care hospices is their economy: One program in San Rafael, California, with only eight of its 54 workers paid full time, cared for 550 patients in five years.

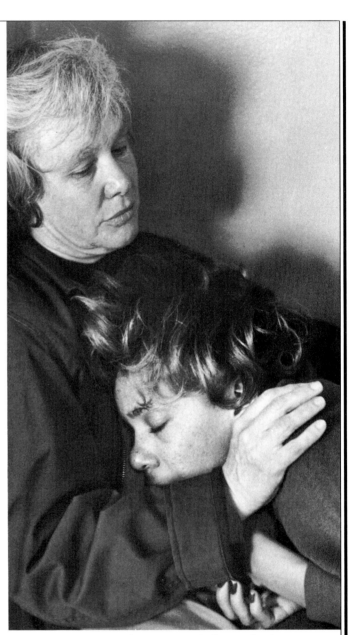

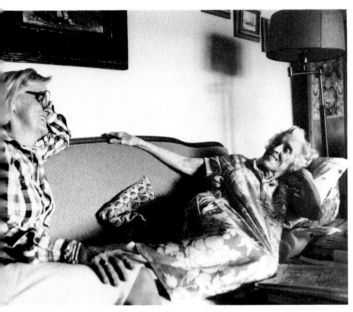

Reclining comfortably in her Washington, D.C., apartment, a patient in her eighties enjoys a visit from a hospice nurse. Most patients and their families cope admirably at home, knowing that hospice nurses are on call at any hour for an emergency.

A hospice volunteer consoles a woman who has just lost her sister to cancer. Hospice staff may work with a bereaved family for up to a year after the patient's death. ''When we take on a patient,'' said one hospice doctor, ''we take on the whole family.''

(only two cited health as the reason). Of those who were still with the company, 10 had served for more than 10 years and 31 had worked for periods ranging from six months to five years. The study concluded: "Cancer-history employees leave their jobs at the same rate as noncancer employees," and "the selective employment of persons with cancer history, in positions for which they are physically qualified, is a sound industrial practice."

These positive conclusions were reached after evaluation of some negative findings. The absence record of the study group, for example, was slightly higher than average. Other studies have shown that as many as half of all fully recovered cancer patients encounter at least one work problem related to their illness, and that up to 10 per cent are temporarily or permanently denied participation in employer-sponsored health insurance plans. In such situations, cancer patients should know that they have some legal recourse. In many places job discrimination against disabled persons—including cancer patients—is forbidden by law. In California, cancer is singled out for legislation. That state specifically prohibits discrimination against "any health impairment related to or associated with a diagnosis of cancer, for which a person has been rehabilitated or cured based on competent medical evidence."

A job is important to most people partly for the direction and purpose it gives their lives, but mainly for income. Cancer is an expensive disease. In much of the industrialized world the direct medical outlay for physicians, hospitals and drugs is paid by governmental health services; in the United States, insurance plans, directly or indirectly subsidized by the government, cover most of this expense for most people. But the economic costs of cancer extend beyond direct medical expense, and everywhere in the world the money to pay for them must be found by the individual.

A cancer patient and his family must expect a drain on financial resources. Neither employers nor insurance plans fully pay the cost of long absences from a job. There are indirect financial problems in protracted treatment far from home—the cost of going to the cancer center, a cost that may recur for months or years; and when the patient is a child, the cost of having a parent accompany him. To meet such demands, many members of a family may have to rally to provide support.

When treatment fails

Coping with cancer is a family affair, of course, from the moment the disease is suspected through the stages of diagnosis and treatment. But this is never more true than when cancer victims cannot return to work or school, and when further hospital treatment would serve no medical purpose. In these circumstances many patients prefer to go home, where they can enjoy constant, loving care from the family.

Because home care of a terminally ill patient is demanding, an increasingly common alternative to the hospital is the hospice *(pages 152-154)*, where medical attention is constantly available but the routine of a hospital is suspended and, as far as possible, patients live the same kind of life they would at home. If a patient craves yogurt or a special brand of Scotch, his tastes are indulged. There are no strict visiting hours; relatives and friends come and go as they please, and even pets can call on the patients.

Hospices, effective home care—indeed, all the strategies for coping with cancer—make death, if it does occur, much easier to bear. At the same time they ennoble the lives of all the participants. Patients and family members who have faced cancer squarely and fought it valiantly and intelligently—and who have secured lengthy and happy remissions—find that the struggle has a value in itself.

"When the possibility of death is on one's mind," wrote television news reporter Betty Rollin about her own battle against cancer, "the problems of life, no matter how great or how niggling, loom less large." Her own treatment was eventually successful, but her account of it, set down while she was still passing through grim cycles of remission and relapse, speaks for all cancer patients, everywhere. "When things go well nowadays," she wrote, "I feel as happy as I ever felt before the operation. When things go badly, I definitely suffer less. A personal hurt, a screw-up at work—such things bother me less now, much less." For Betty Rollin, as for so many, fighting cancer enhanced the value of life. ❋

Generals of the cancer war

"There is a 'looking-under-rocks' aspect to cancer research," said Dr. Lewis Thomas, President of Memorial Sloan-Kettering Cancer Center in New York. "Scientists are still looking for what to look for."

This thesis is borne out by the diversity of research now under way around the world. The war against cancer—an enemy with many faces—is world-wide. It deploys thousands of the scientific community's brightest, best-trained specialists and billions of dollars. Each country's cancer campaigns, its particular ways of looking under particular rocks, reflect that nation's unique skills and theories, even its prevalent cancers. The Japanese, for example, have turned their great talent for technology to developing better diagnostic devices. One result is an endoscope that looks inside the body and provides a three-dimensional image of an organ—especially helpful in detecting cancer of the stomach,

which afflicts the Japanese more than any other people *(page 13)*.

Although nearly every nation is allied in the war on cancer, some of the hardest-fought battles are being waged in the Soviet Union, India, France, Italy, Great Britain, Japan and the United States. Their results are shared directly through bilateral agreements and through organizations such as the International Union against Cancer, headed by Italy's Dr. Umberto Veronesi and headquartered in Geneva, Switzerland. Some cancer experts practically commute on a regular basis from country to country to exchange the latest intelligence from the battle fronts. The variety of efforts and results they report advance the campaign. Observed Dr. Vincent DeVita, of America's National Cancer Institute, one of many generals in the world war against cancer, "If they practice medicine differently in a different country, then you can learn from the difference."

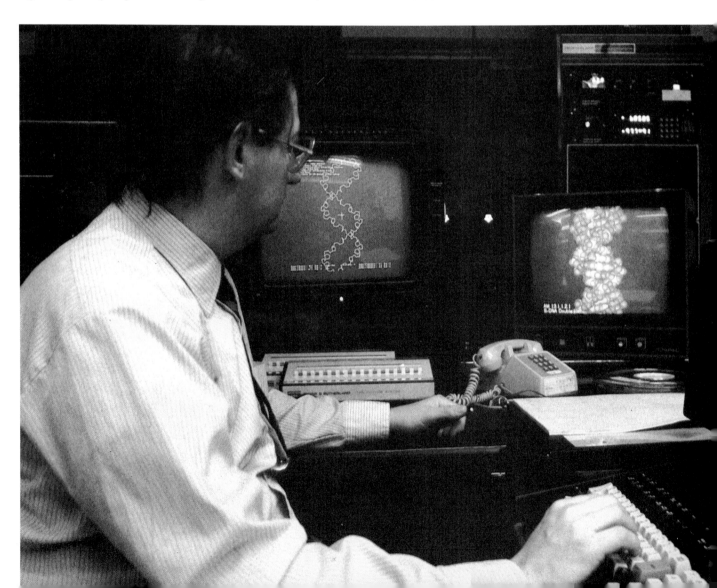

United States: exploiting the new biology

An annual budget of one billion dollars gives the National Cancer Institute 10 times the funds of any other cancer-research organization in the Western countries and makes it a major source of support for laboratories around the world. Among the most promising of NCI's diverse efforts is the use of computers to trace the single genetic aberration that underlies a specific cancer. Progress already made supports the pride of NCI's director, Dr. Vincent T. DeVita Jr. *(right),* who said, ''I'm satisfied that we've made the point that we can cure cancer.''

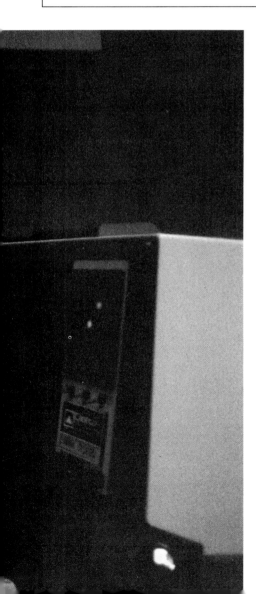

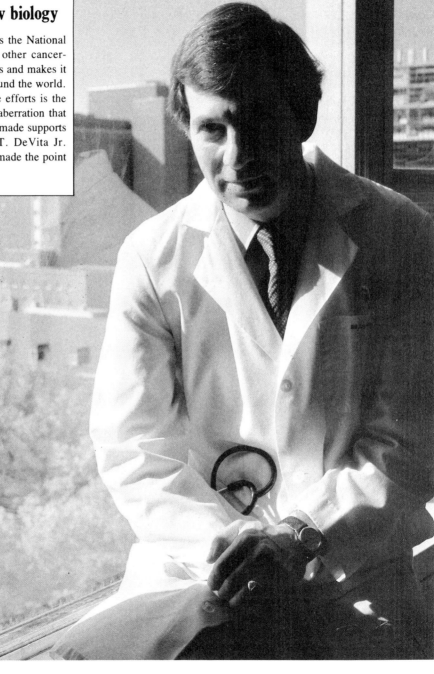

Retrieving computer-stored information with the terminal at right, a scientist constructs video images of DNA (background)— the genetic blueprint for the body—in research for the National Cancer Institute. Computer-simulated rearrangements of DNA provide clues to cancer multiplication.

U.S.S.R.: centralized research

The largest cancer research center in the world covers three city blocks in Moscow. The $180 million center has a staff of 4,000, 59 departments, and beds for 1,000 patients. Directed by Dr. Nikolai Blokhin *(right),* the center oversees the work of 21 regional cancer institutes and clinics, involving doctors and researchers in numbers unequaled elsewhere. Dr. Blokhin believes "it is very important to cultivate in young doctors the desire to retain the human traditions of past medicine. But doctors must also be urged to learn everything new that can be used in diagnosing and treating disease."

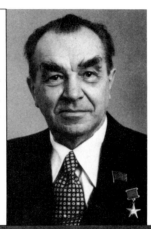

Doctors at Moscow's Cancer Research Center confer at the bedside of a child (below). Most of the 1,000 patients here are treated in clinical trials of new procedures; more routine treatment is provided by 250 other specialized cancer hospitals —four times the number of cancer hospitals in the United States.

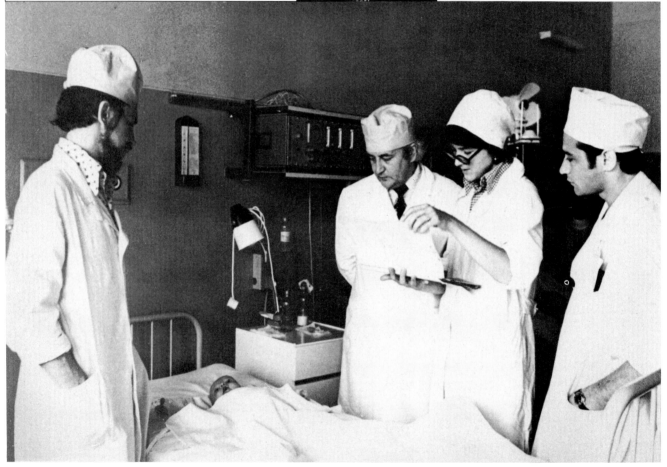

India: studying dangerous habits

The Indian subcontinent offers a case study in cancers caused by such entrenched habits as chewing betel leaf and lime *(page 14),* and smoking with the lighted cigarette end in the mouth. Prevention is the ideal, said Dr. Profulla Desai *(below),* director of Bombay's Tata Memorial Hospital. But for now, India's primary aim—as in much of the Third World—is finding out who is susceptible and how and where these cancers develop. In India, the treatment of cancer remains a secondary concern, for, as Dr. Desai observed sadly, ''Most Indians don't live long enough to get cancer.''

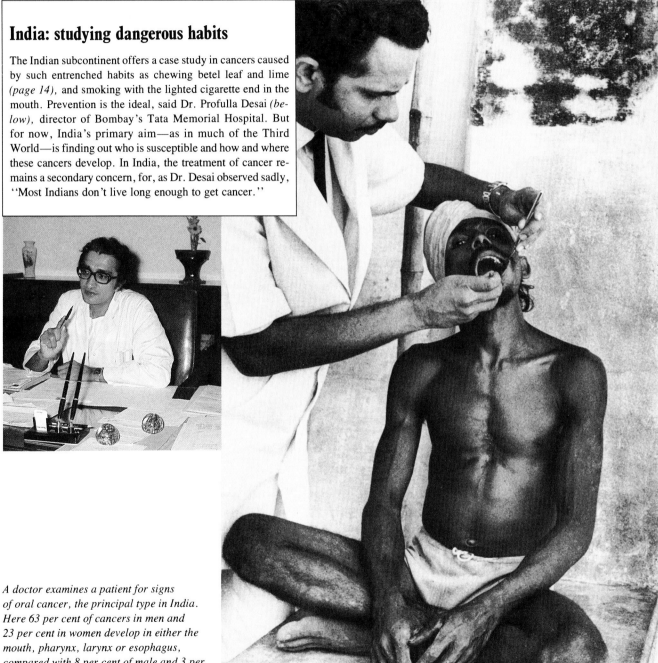

A doctor examines a patient for signs of oral cancer, the principal type in India. Here 63 per cent of cancers in men and 23 per cent in women develop in either the mouth, pharynx, larynx or esophagus, compared with 8 per cent of male and 3 per cent of female cancer victims in America.

Japan: advances through technology

Not surprisingly, Japan is in the forefront in the development of devices for cancer diagnosis and treatment. It supplies doctors around the world with instruments, like the one at right, that enable doctors to see inside the body. But treatment and clinical research as well as technology are the concern of the National Cancer Center. It is directed by Dr. Shichiro Ishikawa *(below)*, a practicing surgeon who involves himself in the care of the center's patients—for each case 10 or more specialists may be allocated, including surgeons, chemotherapists and radiation therapists.

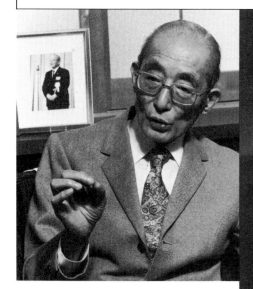

Made in Japan, the instrument in the hands of National Cancer Center surgeon Shigeto Ikeda is a bronchoscope, which can be threaded into a patient's lungs so that a doctor can look for tumors. It is one of many new types developed in Japan to explore the breathing and digestive systems. One gives three-dimensional views; another is connected to a laser, whose powerful beam of light can burn away an internal tumor without surgery.

France: pursuing individual ideas

In France, cancer scientists are urged to solve what Professor Raymond Latarjet *(right)* of the French National League Against Cancer called "enigmas that impassion them." Research there, he said, "has never been really directed," although he made clear that support goes to "those places where we know good work is being done." Instead of emphasizing any one area, he contended, "it is better to leave good people free to go their way and see what will come out." To that end the League awards 50 annual fellowships to scientists under the age of 30 to pursue their interests.

Typical of many French scientists working independently in one of 50 laboratories and receiving special funds for cancer research is this chemist, who is studying the reproductive activity of cancer cells. In a decade, League fellowships sponsored the work of about 500 such young people.

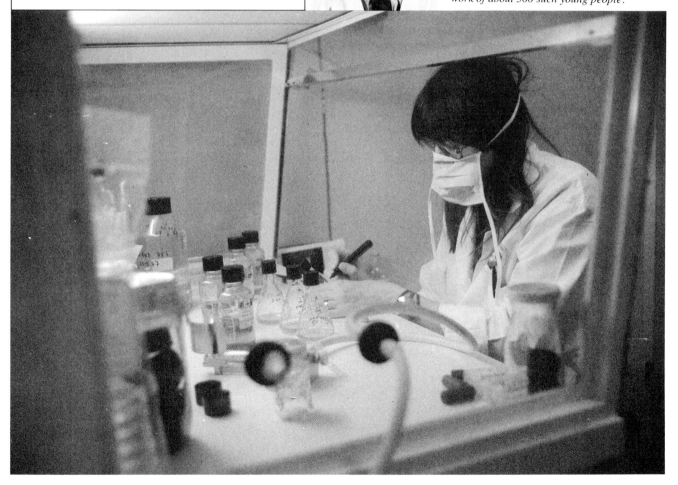

Britain: on the frontier

Unlike most countries, where one governing body oversees cancer research, Britain wages a decentralized battle that is conducted by three separate organizations: the Imperial Cancer Research Fund, the Medical Research Council and the Cancer Research Campaign. The fight is coordinated, however, by a committee under the chairmanship of Sir Alastair Currie *(below)* to ensure, he explained, "that cancer research throughout Britain is properly integrated to avoid duplication of effort." Some of their most promising projects are experiments with drugs that enhance radiation therapy *(right)*.

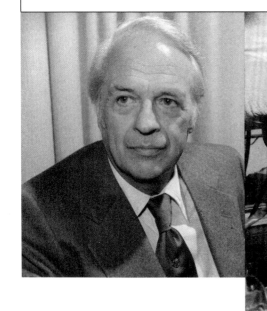

At the Institute of Cancer Research in London, Dr. E. Martin Fielden (left) and Professor G. E. Adams irradiate cells treated with a drug that helps X-rays kill cancers faster. The drug selectively heightens vulnerability to radiation in the cells of the tumor, but not in cells of the surrounding healthy tissue.

Still performing surgery two or three mornings a week, Dr. Umberto Veronesi (below, with a member of his staff) also shoulders dual leadership responsibilities. He is not only director of Italy's major cancer institute but, moreover, serves as president of the International Union against Cancer.

Italy: putting research into practice

Italy's National Cancer Institute aims, says its director, Dr. Umberto Veronesi, "to translate into practice, in a very direct way, results from the laboratory." In 1969, for example, when an Italian pharmaceutical company discovered a microorganism with medical potential on the shores of the Adriatic Sea, samples were brought at once to the cancer institute in Milan. The drug developed from these cultures was tested against tumors in animals, then on patients. Today, the drug—called Adriamycin, after its place of discovery—is used in treating a wide range of malignant tumors.

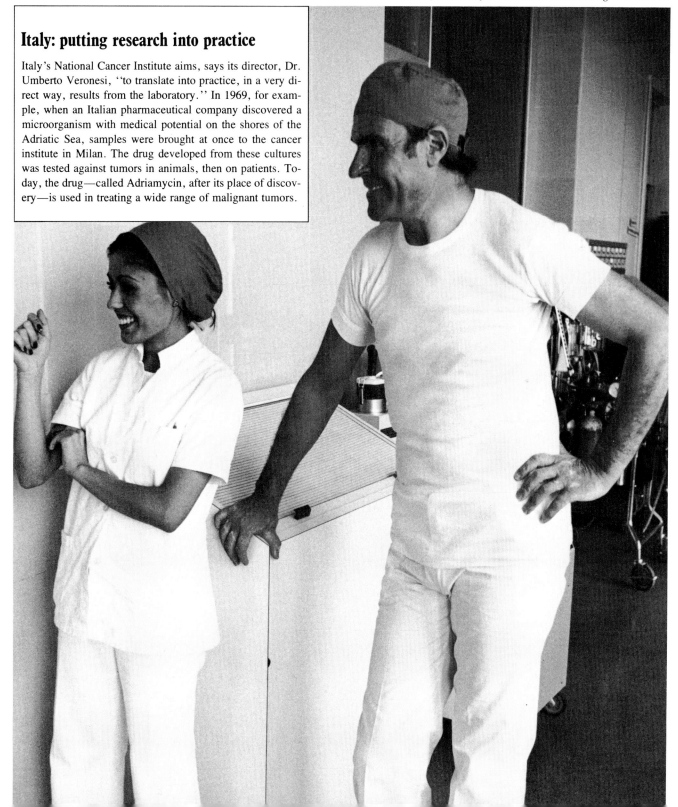

An encyclopedia of symptoms

Most cancers—there are more than 100 types—signal their presence at the early stage, when they are readily cured. But you must recognize the warning yourself, for the first indications are generally painless and may seem inconsequential, not worth bothering a doctor about—barely noticeable bleeding, a strange lump or persistent coughing. By the time major symptoms of serious illness appear, cancer generally has spread so much it is difficult to eradicate. The most common signs of cancer are described below, listed alphabetically. The diseases that may cause each symptom—or, more often, each group of symptoms—are named in small capital letters. Because the early signs of cancer are common and minor, they can also indicate other ailments; the most frequently encountered of these are described as well.

The descriptions given here are simplified. If you notice a symptom that could suggest cancer, consult a doctor even if you are doubtful of the symptom's meaning. Call him immediately; although a cancer symptom does not require treatment in a hospital emergency clinic, delay can be dangerous.

ABDOMINAL PAIN. Pains in the stomach or lower abdomen, among the most common medical complaints of humankind, rarely signal anything worse than a transitory digestive problem. But if the pains are intense or sharp, or if they last more than 48 hours, or if other symptoms are present, get medical attention.

● **Pain in the upper abdomen** occasionally indicates cancer.

If sharp pain under the left ribs is aggravated by breathing, and if it occurs with tenderness in the breastbone area, weakness, fatigue, loss of appetite and weight and unusual bruising, LEUKEMIA, or blood cancer, may be indicated.

If upper abdominal pain is persistent, becomes worse after eating and is accompanied by nausea, vomiting, anemia and weight loss, the problem may be CANCER OF THE STOMACH.

● **Pain in the mid-abdomen** that is crampy and intermittent or that is accompanied by darkish stools and anemia may indicate CANCER OF THE SMALL INTESTINE.

● **Pain in the lower abdomen** can indicate several types of cancer.

If lower abdominal pain is accompanied by blood and mucus in the stool, the problem may be POLYPS, generally benign growths, on the lining of the intestines. Sometimes abdominal cramping and diarrhea occur as well. Consult a physician promptly, for POLYPS can turn cancerous.

If lower abdominal pain in a woman is persistent, and in later stages is accompanied by swelling of the abdomen, weight loss and anemia, CANCER OF THE OVARY may be indicated.

Pain in a man's lower abdomen, groin or scrotum and a mass in the scrotum may signal TESTICULAR CANCER. Urination difficulties are often a sign as well.

If lower abdominal pain is intermittent and appears with bowel changes—blood or mucus in the stools—the condition may indicate CANCER OF THE COLON.

● **Generalized abdominal pain that is variable and that extends to the back or chest,** or that is relieved by sitting up or bending forward, may suggest CANCER OF THE PANCREAS. Nausea, dark urine and pale stools, yellow skin, loss of appetite and weight also signal this cancer.

APPETITE LOSS. Temporary appetite loss is generally due to nothing more than stress or minor illness.

If appetite loss in a child is sudden and is accompanied by fever, nausea, vomiting and a perceptible lump in the abdomen, it may be the result of WILMS' TUMOR, a cancer of the kidney that is curable in about 50 per cent of the cases.

If appetite loss is accompanied by fatigue, pallor, tenderness in the breastbone or abdominal discomfort, it could indicate CHRONIC LYMPHOCYTIC LEUKEMIA or CHRONIC MYELOCYTIC LEUKEMIA.

If appetite loss is accompanied by itching, profuse sweating at night and swelling of the glands in the neck, armpits and groin, HODGKIN'S DISEASE, a cancer of the lymph glands, could be at fault.

If appetite loss is accompanied by a newfound, intense dislike of certain foods or by stomach pains shortly after eating, it may suggest CANCER OF THE STOMACH.

BACK PAIN. Pain in the back is usually due to MUSCLE STRAIN from lifting a heavy object, or from twisting or bending the body in the wrong way. But if back pain occurs with other symptoms, it could indicate other and more serious medical problems.

● **Back pain that is persistent** and occurs with pain in the chest or pelvic area can indicate MULTIPLE MYELOMA, a cancer of the bone marrow. Repeated or constant infections, weakness and weight loss may accompany the other symptoms. Multiple myeloma usually strikes people over 40.

● **Back pain that occurs with a swollen abdomen and bloody urine** may indicate KIDNEY CANCER. Sometimes a lump can be felt. Weight loss and anemia are other symptoms.

● **Back pain that occurs in a man and is accompanied by bloody urine** may also be a symptom of PROSTATE CANCER. Urination may be progressively difficult, painful and frequent, or the stream may be diminished.

● **Back pain that extends to the upper abdomen** and is accompanied by indigestion, brownish urine, pale stools, jaundice and weight loss may suggest PANCREATIC CANCER.

● **Back pain that occurs with bloody vaginal discharge,** irregular periods, or bleeding after intercourse or exertion may indicate CER-VICAL CANCER. Other symptoms may include urinary problems, weight loss or rectal bleeding.

BEHAVIOR CHANGES. Behavior changes, either radical or subtle, can indicate anything from simple insomnia to the brain damage caused by a stroke, but they can also arise from cancer.

● **Behavior changes accompanied by severe headaches,** muscle weakness and disturbances in balance, sight and smell may be caused by a benign or malignant BRAIN TUMOR. Convulsions, fatigue, sleepiness and poor mental functioning may also occur in the later stages of the disease.

● **Behavior changes accompanied by muscle weakness restricted to one side of the body** and any or all of the symptoms listed above may indicate a generalized BRAIN CANCER.

BLEEDING. *(See also: BLOOD IN STOOL, URINE CHANGES AND URINA-TION DIFFICULTIES and VAGINAL BLEEDING AND DISCHARGE).* Unexpected or excess bleeding can signal a number of medical conditions—vitamin deficiencies, circulatory disorders such as high blood pressure, genetic blood diseases such as HEMOPHILIA and, in women, menstrual complications. Most instances of excess or unexplainable bleeding require medical attention, but only a few are related to cancer.

If persistent oral bleeding is accompanied by bloody mucus and choking attacks, the cause may be CANCER OF THE THYROID. Other indications are a swelling on the front of the neck, hoarseness, difficulty swallowing and speaking, and weight loss.

If oral bleeding occurs with small white patches inside the mouth, it could suggest CANCER OF THE MOUTH. Stiffness in the jaw and pain in the mouth or jaw are other symptoms.

● **Bleeding from the nose** rarely signals anything more serious than the rupture of a tiny blood vessel, but if frequent nosebleeds occur with other symptoms, inform your doctor.

If frequent nosebleeds are accompanied by acute pain in the nose, by suddenly nasal speech, or by a feeling of fullness in the nose, the cause may be CANCER OF THE PHARYNX, the tube that connects the mouth with the esophagus.

BLOOD IN STOOL. Bloody or darkened stools can indicate dozens of ailments, from comparatively minor problems such as HEM-ORRHOIDS—ruptured veins near the anus—to life-threatening diseases such as COLON CANCER. If the blood is red, it indicates an ailment in the lower intestine; if the stool is dark—almost black—the source of the blood is higher in the digestive tract.

If rectal bleeding occurs without pain or any other symptoms, it may come from a POLYP, or small growth, in the colon. Although these growths are usually benign, certain types may lead to cancer. Consult a physician.

If bloody stools are accompanied by mucus, by chronic constipation alternating with thin and watery diarrhea, by narrow stools or by pain in the rectum and chronic fatigue, CANCER OF THE RECTUM may be indicated. Sometimes a lump can be felt near the anus.

If bloody stools occur with mucus, with a persistent change in the size, color or number of stools, or with intermittent pain in the lower abdomen, the problem may be CANCER OF THE COLON. Other signs of colon cancer are weakness and weight loss or the presence of blood in the stool.

If darkened stools occur with intermittent cramps in the mid-abdomen, weakness, pallor, and weight loss, CANCER OF THE SMALL INTESTINE may be the cause.

If darkened stools occur with a feeling of fullness, nausea and pressure in the upper abdomen, belching, heartburn after meals, and loss of appetite, CANCER OF THE STOMACH may be indicated. Pallor, fatigue, weight loss, diarrhea and vomiting of blood may also occur with this cancer.

BONE PAIN. Bone pain can point to any of several ailments, including OSTEOARTHRITIS and a disintegrative bone disorder called OSTEOPOROSIS, which primarily affects elderly women. But bone pain can signal cancer, especially if other symptoms are present.

If bone pain is persistent and is followed or accompanied by swelling of the painful area, the cause may be CANCER OF THE BONE. The most common areas for bone cancer are legs, thighs, shoulders and hips, and it most frequently strikes adolescents.

If bone pain is deep and penetrating, and if it is worse after exertion, the problem may be MULTIPLE MYELOMA, a cancer of the bone marrow. Spontaneous fractures are common with this disease, as is anemia. Thighs, pelvis and upper arms are the most common sites for this cancer.

BOWEL HABIT CHANGES. An abrupt change in bowel habits—particularly if it represents a persisting alteration of a previously regular pattern—can be a warning of serious illness, including several cancers, if it cannot be readily explained by minor illness or modifications in diet or life style.

● **Constipation with abdominal pain that extends to the back** and is relieved by sitting up or bending forward may be due to CANCER OF THE PANCREAS. Yellow skin, clay-colored stools, diarrhea, appetite loss, vomiting and the vomiting of blood are other signs of this cancer.

● **Constipation that alternates with diarrhea** and is accompanied by thin, ribbon-like stools or by blood in the stool may suggest

CANCER OF THE SMALL INTESTINE. Other symptoms are rectal discomfort that is not relieved by a bowel movement, pain in the rectum, abdominal cramps and chronic flatulence.

BREAST DISCHARGE. A clear or bloody fluid issuing from a woman's nipple may indicate either benign or malignant tumors. Because cancer is a possibility, see a doctor as soon as possible.

BREAST LUMPS: *see LUMPS*

BRUISES. Bruises are produced by bleeding that takes place under the skin. They usually result from minor injuries and can take the familiar black-and-blue appearance, or can appear as brownish spots or small reddish areas. Only if you bruise extremely easily, or if you notice bruises or small purplish, reddish or brown areas that cannot be accounted for, do they require a physician's attention.

If small bruises or reddish or purplish spots appear on the skin, or if a bruised, black-and-blue appearance is present, ACUTE LEUKEMIA may be the cause. This serious but curable form of blood cancer strikes children more often than adults. Other signs include frequent and persistent infections, high fever, joint pain and pallor.

CHANGE IN BLADDER HABITS: *See URINE CHANGES AND URINATION DIFFICULTIES*
CHANGE IN BOWEL HABITS: *See BOWEL HABIT CHANGES*
CHANGE IN MOLE OR WART: *See MOLE AND WART CHANGES*

CHEST PAIN. Chest pain is common and can arise from causes as diverse as indigestion and muscle strain and as serious as heart disease and cancer. Few chest pains indicate a life-threatening condition, and fewer still cancer. Only if the pains appear with other, specific symptoms might cancer be indicated.

If pain under the breastbone is accompanied by weight loss, thirst, dehydration, flatulence and heavy salivation, CANCER OF THE ESOPHAGUS may be the cause.

If the chest pain occurs with blood-streaked phlegm and wheezing, the cause may be LUNG CANCER. Breathing problems, weakness and weight loss are other signs of this disease.

If the chest pain occurs with prolonged weakness, MULTIPLE MYELOMA, a cancer of the bone marrow, may be indicated. Other signs are persistent infections, weight loss and sometimes pain in the back or pelvis.

CONVULSIONS. A convulsion is always a sign of a serious medical problem. Consult a doctor immediately. The best-known cause of convulsions is EPILEPSY, a disorder of the nervous system that produces seizures characterized by clenched fists, twitching muscles, jerking arms and legs and incontinence. A person with these symptoms should see a physician as soon as possible.

● **Convulsions accompanied by severe headaches,** dizziness and vomiting may indicate a benign or malignant BRAIN TUMOR. Such a tumor may produce other symptoms that depend on its location.

COUGHING. Coughing is the body's attempt to clear fluids, mucus, dust and allergy-causing substances from the lungs or throat. Although coughing usually indicates a minor irritation or respiratory infection, a persistent cough may suggest a more serious condition and demands prompt medical attention.

● **A cough that persists** may point to LUNG CANCER, especially if it occurs with wheezing, bloody phlegm, hoarseness and difficulty in swallowing. Secondary symptoms include swelling of the finger tips, arms or legs, chest pain or a tingling sensation in the arms.

DIZZINESS (Vertigo). Ear problems, from wax in the ear to a PERFORATED EARDRUM, may cause dizziness. But if dizziness occurs with certain other symptoms, any of several types of cancer could be indicated.

If dizziness occurs with loss of balance, problems of sight, hearing and smell, hallucinations, and disturbances of memory or thinking, a BRAIN TUMOR may be the cause. Other signs include frequent or severe headaches, vomiting, muscle weakness, lethargy, convulsions and sudden bizarre behavior.

EYE CHANGES. An eye may abruptly change appearance, becoming reddened, swollen and teary if a foreign object becomes lodged in it or if the person has an infection or allergy. But some eye changes may indicate that a tumor is present.

If a child's pupil becomes whitish or the eyeball enlarges, the cause may be RETINOBLASTOMA, a cancer of the eye. Other symptoms include squinting and sudden vision impairment.

FATIGUE. If fatigue is not relieved by rest and relaxation, or if it is accompanied by other symptoms, it needs medical attention.

● **Fatigue coupled with tenderness in the breastbone** area may signal CHRONIC MYELOCYTIC LEUKEMIA, a blood cancer that mainly affects adults. Appetite loss, weakness, weight loss and heaviness or discomfort in the upper abdomen may accompany this disease.

● **Fatigue** can signal another type of blood cancer, CHRONIC LYMPHOCYTIC LEUKEMIA. In that ailment, paleness and swelling of the lymph glands in the neck may also occur.

● **Fatigue accompanied by personality changes,** poor sensory powers, loss of balance, drowsiness or vomiting may indicate CANCER OF THE BRAIN. The symptoms vary widely, depending on where in the brain the tumor is located. Other possible signs of this condition are headache, weakness and poor mental functioning.

FEVER. Body temperature above normal (98.6° F.) is not by itself a primary indication of cancer, but it can be a secondary signal when other symptoms are present or when it lasts more than three days.

HEADACHES. The vast majority of headaches result from tension or adverse mood states such as depression, from a cold or flu, from eyestrain or from taking certain medications, including oral contraceptives. Intense, persistent headaches, however, especially if other symptoms are present, demand medical attention.
● **Prolonged severe headaches** may signal the presence of a benign or malignant BRAIN TUMOR, especially when accompanied by muscle weakness, drowsiness, lack of coordination, personality changes and sensory disorders.

HOARSENESS. Common infections such as a cold or influenza may cause hoarseness, as may overuse of your voice. Hoarseness also may be due to ACUTE LARYNGITIS, an inflammation of the voice box. If any hoarseness persists for more than 10 days, have a checkup, for the condition can indicate a more serious ailment.
● **Prolonged hoarseness** can signal POLYPS (benign growths) on the vocal cords or CANCER OF THE LARYNX—the voice box.
● **Prolonged hoarseness coupled with a chronic cough,** chest pain, wheezing and breathing difficulty might indicate LUNG CANCER. Fever and loss of weight may also occur.
● **Prolonged hoarseness plus pressure or pain under the breastbone** may indicate CANCER OF THE ESOPHAGUS. Constant thirst, chronic belching, coughing and loss of weight are other signals.

INDIGESTION. Indigestion is seldom serious unless it is prolonged, recurrent or severe, or unless other symptoms are present.
● **Persistent or severe indigestion with weight loss,** a sudden distaste for certain foods or a feeling of fullness after eating small portions may indicate STOMACH CANCER. Blackish stools and the vomiting of blood are other symptoms.

INFECTIONS. Most of the time, an infection is just that—an infection and nothing more. But any infection, however minor it may seem, should be discussed with a physician. And repeated or persistent infections, especially if other symptoms are present, may

signal any of several types of cancer: Some cancers depress the body's defense system, leaving it vulnerable to infection.

ITCHING. Most itching occurs because of SKIN IRRITATION, an ALLERGY or a RASH. Only when it is intense and prolonged, or when it occurs with other symptoms, might it indicate a truly serious ailment such as cancer.
If intense itching is accompanied by painful enlargement of the lymph glands in the neck, armpits or groin, and if it occurs with night sweating, fever, fatigue, weakness, and loss of appetite and weight, the cause of these symptoms may be HODGKIN'S DISEASE or LYMPHOMA, two cancers of the lymph system. Swelling on one side of the neck is more apt to indicate HODGKIN'S DISEASE; swelling on both sides, LYMPHOMA.

JOINT PAIN. The cause of joint pain is usually easy to discern—the pain is from an injury such as a sprained ankle or a twisted knee. But persistent joint pain whose cause is not easily discerned can be an indication of debilitating and serious illnesses such as arthritis and cancer.
● **Joint pain with high fever** and small reddish or purple spots on or under the skin may suggest ACUTE LEUKEMIA. Repeated infections, a bruised appearance, abdominal pain, blood in the urine or feces, or bleeding from the nose or mouth are other symptoms.

LUMP. A lump anywhere in the body is one of the most important signs of cancer. Fortunately, few lumps are malignant. Most are CYSTS, or benign tumors, swellings that rarely pose a threat. But if you should notice a lump or thickening of tissue anywhere on your body, or if you notice any sort of unaccountable swelling, do not diagnose it yourself. See a doctor within a day or so.
● **The most commonly discovered lumps are those of the breast.** Most are benign, but you should take no chances: Make an appointment for a breast examination promptly. In most instances, the doctor can feel the lump and make an educated guess as to whether it is benign or malignant.
If the lump is firm and well defined, and if it feels like rubber and can be moved about within the breast, chances are that it is a FIBROADENOMA, a benign tumor.
If the lump is small, painless and not easily moved within the breast, or if it occurs with thickening or dimpling of the breast skin, BREAST CANCER is a more distinct possibility. There may be detectable changes in the breast contour and a retraction of or discharge from the nipple as well.
● **Lumps of the neck area** can be highly significant and should be

reported to your doctor. However, like breast lumps, most of them are not cancerous.

If a painless neck lump is located in the center of the neck and occurs with difficulty swallowing and speaking, with weight loss and bloody mucus, CANCER OF THE THYROID could be the cause.

If painless neck lumps are on one or both sides of the neck, and are accompanied by itching, fatigue, weakness, pallor, loss of weight and difficulty breathing, HODGKIN'S DISEASE or certain LYMPHOMAS, cancers of the lymph system, could be the cause. In HODGKIN'S DISEASE, the neck lumps usually are found only on one side of the neck; in LYMPHOMA, on both sides. Repeated or persistent fevers and swelling of the lymph glands under the arms and in the groin may accompany the other symptoms.

If painless neck lumps occur in a child and are accompanied by frequent bruising, the appearance of red spots under the skin, or by bleeding from the mouth or nose, LEUKEMIA may be indicated. Other indications are blood in the stool or urine, pain in the joints and abdomen, fever and fatigue.

If the painful swelling in the neck is accompanied by difficulty swallowing, and if opening the mouth is accompanied by earache and pain radiating to the side of the face, CANCER OF THE PHARYNX or CANCER OF THE THROAT may be the cause. Speech may sound nasal and there may be nosebleeds as well.

● **Small, pearly, raised lumps just under the skin** may signal SKIN CANCER. Such lumps can become ulcerated and raw, but if they are treated properly and promptly, this development can be avoided. Skin cancer can almost always be cured.

● **Lumps in the abdomen** can point to several different ailments, few of them cancers but most requiring medical attention.

If the abdominal lump occurs with pain that radiates from the abdomen to the back, CANCER OF THE KIDNEYS may be the cause. Such a lump may occur alone, or it may be accompanied by a lump in the middle of the back. Other signs are blood in the urine, fatigue and weight loss. Similar symptoms in a child may indicate WILMS' TUMOR, a kidney cancer of youngsters.

● **Lumps in the pelvic region** are always worth reporting to a doctor, for many common cancers are located there.

If a woman's pelvic lump occurs with difficulty urinating, with heavy menstrual bleeding, and with pain in the region, a BENIGN FIBROID TUMOR OF THE UTERUS may be the cause. Large lumps may be felt in the abdomen as well.

If a woman's pelvic lump is associated with abdominal pain and swelling, backache and vaginal bleeding, the problem may be CANCER OF THE OVARY. Other indications are changes in urinary or bowel habits and enlarged and painful breasts. A BENIGN TUMOR OF THE OVARY may present similar symptoms, often accompanied by cessation of the normal menstrual periods and development of such masculine characteristics as a deeper voice and facial hair.

If a man's pelvic lump is located in his scrotum, he most likely has a CYST but the problem could be CANCER OF THE TESTES, a fast-growing cancer that mainly affects young men. There may be scrotal pain as well.

MOLE AND WART CHANGES. Almost everyone has a few moles—flat or raised dark spots on the skin—and many people have warts, the pigmented skin growths caused by a virus. Although warts and moles are generally harmless by themselves, those that are chronically irritated may change and give rise to a virulent form of skin cancer called MALIGNANT MELANOMA.

If a wart or mole seems to grow or change color, shape, texture or consistency, consult a physician. It may become firmer or harder all over or at the edges, somewhat bumpy on the surface, inflamed, painful, moist or ulcerated, or it may begin to bleed without cause. The borders of a flat, darkish mole may become fuzzy, irregular or notched, and small dark spots may appear around it. A raised mole may become uniformly bluish black, bluish gray or bluish red or develop a white "halo" around it. A new mole that develops in adulthood should also be seen by a doctor; black or dark brown raised growths that appear suddenly are the most suspicious.

MOUTH AND LIP SORES. Most mouth and lip sores are COLD SORES or FEVER BLISTERS, due to a viral infection, and heal of themselves. Two types of sores, however, may be signs of cancer.

● **A sore on the lips** that does not heal and bleeds easily may be caused by CANCER OF THE LIP.

● **A sore in the mouth** that does not heal after two weeks, may begin as a soft, white patch that thickens and hardens, and may be accompanied by a burning sensation is a possible sign of CANCER OF THE MOUTH.

NAUSEA AND VOMITING. Nausea—the feeling that one may vomit at any moment—and vomiting itself are symptoms of a great variety of illnesses, mainly not related to cancer. The most common cause is ordinary INDIGESTION, which usually comes on immediately after eating and may be accompanied by heartburn, a feeling of fullness, belching, abdominal distress and passing of gas; all of these usually subside after a few hours. Nausea and vomiting that is persistent and severe, or that occurs with patterns of other symptoms—such as a lump in the abdomen, a persistent loss of appetite, blood in the stool or urine, pain in the back or abdomen, or severe dizziness—demands prompt medical attention. It could signal several cancers that afflict the digestive system or urinary tract.

PAIN: *See ABDOMINAL PAIN, BACK PAIN, BONE PAIN, CHEST PAIN, JOINT PAIN, PROSTATE PAIN and TESTICULAR AND SCROTAL PAIN*

PALENESS. Paleness is a relative term, and many people are naturally pale. However, extreme paleness in the inner part of the eyelid or in the nailbed is a special symptom of a condition doctors call pallor, and continuous pallor is a sign of one type of cancer.

• **Continuous pallor** that is accompanied by swelling of the glands in the neck, weakness, lethargy and loss of appetite may be caused by LEUKEMIA, a blood cancer.

PHLEGM CHANGES. Sticky, heavy mucus in the throat is a common sign of an infection of the upper respiratory tract, but may also indicate one form of cancer.

• **Sticky, heavy mucus that builds gradually** and is accompanied by persistent hoarseness and coughing, earache and breathing difficulties, may be caused by CANCER OF THE LARYNX.

PROSTATE PAIN. Pain in the region of a man's prostate gland—between the scrotum and anus—can suggest any of several medical problems, all worthy of a doctor's attention.

• **Severe pain that occurs between the scrotum and anus,** and radiates to the testes, may suggest CANCER OF THE PROSTATE. The pain may occur with swelling of the prostate, difficult, painful or frequent urination, pain while sitting, chills, fever and occasionally bloody urine. Additional symptoms may include intermittent impotence, premature ejaculation and blood in the semen.

SHORTNESS OF BREATH. Many people experience shortness of breath after physical exertion, after hearty eating or at high altitudes. There is reason for concern, however, when shortness of breath is persistent, is not explained by a readily detectable cause, or is accompanied by other symptoms. In such a case, consult a physician promptly.

If shortness of breath occurs in a child who also has a firm abdominal lump, NEUROBLASTOMA, a childhood cancer of the nervous system, may be the cause. Fever and weight loss may occur as well.

If shortness of breath occurs with persistent coughing that produces bloody sputum, LUNG CANCER may be indicated. Coughing, wheezing, chest pain, weakness and weight loss are other signs.

SKIN SORES. Skin sores in such forms as whiteheads, blackheads and pimples may be caused by ACNE; a doctor can prescribe medication that will lessen these outbreaks. One type of skin sore is a possible sign of cancer.

• **White or red sores** that are raised from the surface and become hard, crusted and ulcerated—that is, marked by the disintegration of tissue and the formation of pus—may be caused by SKIN CANCER. This type of cancer is generally curable.

SORE THROAT. A sore throat is a common symptom of infections ranging from colds and influenza to bronchitis. But a sore throat sometimes gives rise to suspicions of malignant disease.

If a sore throat is accompanied by pain in the throat and ear, the trouble could be CANCER OF THE TONGUE.

If a sore throat occurs with pain that radiates to the side of the face, with difficulty opening the mouth, or with persistent coughing, CANCER OF THE THROAT may be indicated. Lymph glands in the neck may swell in this disease.

If a sore throat occurs with hoarseness, difficulty breathing and swallowing, bad breath, pain in the ear and a constant need to clear the throat, the cause may be CANCER OF THE LARYNX.

If a sore throat occurs with high fever, joint pains, small purplish red spots over the body, paleness, weakness, bleeding from the mouth, or bloody stool or urine, LEUKEMIA may be indicated.

SWALLOWING DIFFICULTIES. A sore throat from a cold may bring on minor problems in swallowing, as may a number of other, more serious ailments, ranging from TONSILLITIS, or inflamed tonsils, to ESOPHAGEAL CANCER.

If swallowing is difficult and painful, or if there is the feeling that food is sticking in the passageway behind the breastbone, CANCER OF THE ESOPHAGUS may be indicated. Dehydration, coughing, flatulence, bad breath, fever and pallor are other signs.

SWEATING. Profuse sweating may occur in any illness that produces high fever, in some types of FOOD POISONING, where it is often combined with nausea, vomiting, and pain in the abdomen, or in cases of HEAT EXHAUSTION, where it may occur with cold skin, headaches, dizziness, nausea and faintness. Get medical help. In such cases, the cause may be easily suspected, but when sweating seems to appear spontaneously and without cause, or when it is accompanied by other symptoms, potentially serious medical conditions may be indicated.

If profuse nighttime sweating occurs with swelling of the lymph glands in the neck, groin or underarms, HODGKIN'S DISEASE, a lymph cancer, may be the cause. Other signs include intense itching, weakness, fever, loss of appetite and weight loss. Another lymph cancer, LYMPHOMA, may cause excessive sweating. Its other symptoms are the same as HODGKIN'S DISEASE, but the swelling may occur on both sides of the neck rather than one.

SWELLING: *See LUMPS*

TESTICULAR AND SCROTAL PAIN. Pain in the testicles and scrotum may be caused by an UNDESCENDED TESTICLE, by URETHRITIS, inflammation of the tube that carries urine from the bladder, or by MUMPS ORCHITIS, inflammation of the testicles by a mumps virus. Only if the pain is accompanied by other symptoms might cancer be indicated.

● **A lump in the scrotum** that increases in size and produces a dull, achy pain may suggest CANCER OF THE TESTES. Testicular pain may occur with pain in the lower abdomen or groin. Feminization may also occur.

THINKING AND MEMORY DIFFICULTIES. A handful of diseases can produce problems of thought and memory, and any such difficulties should be reported to a doctor. Only rarely do thinking and memory difficulties indicate cancer, and only when other symptoms are present.

If mental impairment is combined with nausea, vomiting, lethargy, dizziness, convulsions and severe headache, a malignant or benign BRAIN TUMOR may be the cause. Other symptoms include vision and hearing problems, personality changes or hallucinations.

URINE CHANGES AND URINATION DIFFICULTIES. The composition of the urine can reveal key clues to a person's physical condition, and problems with urination may point to any number of ailments. Thus, any change in urinary habits may be a sign of illness—rarely cancer, but deserving of medical attention.

● **Changes in the color, clarity, quantity or odor of urine** can be a sign of several ailments. Report any such change to your doctor.

If urine suddenly becomes brownish or abnormally dark, and if it is accompanied by pain in the upper abdomen that extends to the back, you may have CANCER OF THE PANCREAS. Other symptoms include pale stools, indigestion, weight loss and yellow skin.

If rust-colored, reddish or bloody urine occurs with pain in the ribs and spine, pallor and a lump in the abdomen, CANCER OF THE KIDNEYS may be the cause. Bloody urine in children may be a symptom of WILMS' TUMOR, a kidney cancer of youngsters. Abdominal swelling is common. Pain, pallor, appetite loss and weight loss also may occur.

If the passage of bloody urine is painless at first, then occurs with pain, it may signal CANCER OF THE BLADDER.

If a man's passage of urine is accompanied by pain from the outset, and if urination becomes progressively more difficult, frequent or urgent, CANCER OF THE PROSTATE may be the cause. Urine output may be scant. Blood in the urine frequently accompanies these symptoms, but it need not be present to indicate cancer.

● **Urinary difficulties**—unusually frequent urination, an abnor-

mally powerful urge to urinate, painful urination and the inability to pass urine—may or may not be accompanied by changes in the urine itself. With or without changes in the urine, such difficulties can indicate a range of ailments.

If a woman's urination becomes increasingly difficult and painful, and if there is any marked change in the pattern of menstrual bleeding, the cause may be a benign tumor in the uterus or CANCER OF THE UTERUS.

If a woman's urination becomes increasingly frequent and urgent, and if it is accompanied by a watery vaginal discharge, by painful defecation, by bleeding or pain after intercourse, CANCER OF THE VAGINA may be indicated.

VAGINAL BLEEDING AND DISCHARGE. A small amount of mucus-like discharge from the vagina at the time of ovulation is a normal occurrence and does not require medical attention. But malodorous, tinted or blood-streaked discharge or bleeding between menstrual periods may indicate a VAGINAL, VULVAR or CERVICAL INFECTION, VENEREAL DISEASE, a HORMONAL IMBALANCE or CANCER OF THE FEMALE REPRODUCTIVE SYSTEM. Report any such discharge to a physician.

If vaginal bleeding starts and stops between regular menstrual periods, or occurs frequently after intercourse or a pelvic examination, CANCER OF THE CERVIX may be indicated. A watery, thin, brownish or malodorous discharge is another common symptom. Other signs are low back pain, hip pain, loss of weight and strength, frequent urination and increased urinary output.

If significant vaginal bleeding occurs within weeks of conception, labor or a miscarriage, the cause may be CHORIOCARCINOMA, a curable cancer affecting the uterus and Fallopian tubes. There may be an unusual vaginal discharge or a feeling of pressure in the groin.

If vaginal discharge is blood-stained or brownish, or if it occurs with swelling and discomfort in the abdomen, CANCER OF THE FALLOPIAN TUBES may be the cause.

If vaginal discharge is offensive in odor or is accompanied by abdominal pain, pain during urination, or pain during intercourse, CANCER OF THE VAGINA may be the cause.

If a thin, watery vaginal discharge occurs with unusual bleeding, itching, or both, CANCER OF THE VULVA may be indicated. Pain may occur in the area.

● **Vaginal bleeding that occurs after menopause** is a significant warning sign of several disorders, notably HORMONAL IMBALANCES and at least two cancers.

If postmenopausal vaginal bleeding starts as a watery, blood-streaked discharge but later contains more blood, CANCER OF THE ENDOMETRIUM may be the cause. The discharge may be thin and sometimes brown-tinged. Gastric pain, low back pain and feelings of abdominal pressure or contraction may occur as well. This cancer is rare but possible among women still having regular periods.

If vaginal bleeding after menopause is accompanied by enlargement of the abdomen, abdominal pain or tenderness, or by severe or persistent indigestion, the cause may be CANCER OF THE OVARY. Backache and difficulty urinating may accompany this disease. Women who have yet to reach menopause should be wary of these symptoms as well, for though the cancer is rare among such women, it can occur.

VISION DISTURBANCES. Sight may be changed in a number of ways: Vision may be blurred, dimmed or distorted, or unaccountable flashes of light, spots or colors may be seen. Any such change should be reported to a doctor, for it could signal such problems as CATARACTS, clouding of the lens of the eye; or GLAUCOMA, a disorder in which pressure within the eye increases. Only if other symptoms are present might cancer be indicated.

● **Headache that occurs with reduced vision** may indicate CANCER OF THE BRAIN. Other possible symptoms are weakness, loss of balance and coordination, personality changes, constant tiredness or sleepiness, nausea and vomiting.

● **Constant squinting and difficulty seeing,** especially in a child, may suggest RETINOBLASTOMA. This cancer of the eye primarily affects children under the age of four and may be signaled by a whitish pupil or an enlargement of the eyeball.

WEAKNESS.

Weakness is a sign of numerous ailments and conditions, from the common cold and influenza to a wide variety of cancers, among them those of the lymph system, nervous system, gall bladder, blood, bones and lungs. Weakness that indicates cancer usually is severe and persistent, and may be accompanied by other symptoms, such as swelling of the lymph glands of the neck, armpits and groin, persistent coughing and infections, or bone and abdominal pain. Report any such weakness to a physician.

WEIGHT LOSS. Loss of weight is a symptom of nearly every cancer. But weight loss, by itself, seldom indicates the disease; other symptoms usually are present when cancer is implicated. Nevertheless, any unaccountable weight loss should be reported to a doctor, whether accompanying symptoms are present or not.

● **Weight loss coupled with difficulties swallowing** may indicate CANCER OF THE THYROID, CANCER OF THE ESOPHAGUS or HODGKIN'S DISEASE, a lymph cancer.

● **Weight loss and chest pain** may point to LUNG CANCER.

● **Weight loss and a penetrating upper abdominal pain** that extends to the back may suggest CANCER OF THE PANCREAS.

● **Weight loss and pain in the upper right abdomen** near the center may be due to CANCER OF THE GALL BLADDER.

● **Weight loss** can be a sign of STOMACH CANCER, especially if it is accompanied by swelling in the abdomen, heartburn, a sudden dislike for certain foods, anemia, vomiting of blood and the passing of black stools.

● **A child who loses weight rapidly** and whose stomach is swollen may have NEUROBLASTOMA, a nerve cancer.

● **Weight loss accompanied by irregular menstrual periods,** bloody vaginal discharge between periods and bleeding after intercourse or upon exertion, may suggest CANCER OF THE CERVIX.

● **Weight loss that occurs with back, chest or pelvic pain,** with weakness and persistent infections may be a sign of MULTIPLE MYELOMA, a cancer of the bone marrow.

Bibliography

BOOKS

Alsop, Stewart, *Stay of Execution*. Lippincott, 1973.

Baker, Lynn S., *You and Leukemia*. W. B. Saunders, 1978.

Brody, Jane E., *You Can Fight Cancer and Win*. Quadrangle/The New York Times Book Company, 1977.

Cairns, John, *Cancer: Science and Society*. W. H. Freeman, 1978.

Del Regato, Juan A., and Harlan J. Spjut, *Ackerman and del Regato's Cancer Diagnosis, Treatment and Prognosis*. C. V. Mosby, 1977.

Epstein, Samuel S., *The Politics of Cancer*. Sierra Club Books, 1978.

Feifel, Herman, ed., *The Meaning of Death*. McGraw-Hill, 1959.

Fraumeni, Joseph F., Jr., *Persons at High Risk of Cancer*. Academic Press, 1975.

Glemser, Bernard, *Mr. Burkitt and Africa*. World Publishing, 1970.

Glucksberg, Harold, and Jack W. Singer, *Cancer Care*. The Johns Hopkins University Press, 1980.

Harris, R.J.C., ed., *What We Know About Cancer*. London: George Allen & Unwin, 1970.

Highland, Joseph H., et al., *Malignant Neglect*. Vintage, 1979.

Ipswitch, Elaine, *Scott Was Here*. Delacorte Press, 1979.

Israël, Lucien, *Conquering Cancer*. Random House, 1978.

Kushner, Rose, *Breast Cancer*. Harcourt Brace Jovanovich, 1975.

LaFond, Richard E., *Cancer—The Outlaw Cell*. American Chemical Society, 1978.

Lee, Laurel, *Walking Through the Fire*. Dutton, 1977.

Levitt, Paul M., and Elissa S. Guralnick, *The Cancer Reference Book*. Paddington Press, 1979.

Milan, Albert R., *Breast Self-Examination*. Workman Publishing, 1980.

Morra, Marion, and Eve Potts, *Choices: Realistic Alternatives in Cancer Treatment*. Avon, 1980.

Order, Stanley E., Joyce Kopicky, and Steven A. Leibel, *Principles of Successful Radiation Therapy*. G. K. Hall, 1979.

Renneker, Mark, and Steven Leib, eds., *Understanding Cancer*. Bull Publishing, 1979.

Rettig, Richard A., *Cancer Crusade*. Princeton University Press, 1977.

Rollin, Betty, *First, You Cry*. Lippincott, 1976.

Rosenbaum, Ernest H., *Living With Cancer*. Praeger, 1975.

Ross, Walter Sanford, *The Climate Is Hope: How They Triumphed Over Cancer*. Prentice-Hall, 1965.

Rossman, Parker, *Hospice*. Fawcett Columbine, 1977.

Ryan, Cornelius, and Kathryn Morgan Ryan, *A Private Battle*. Simon and Schuster, 1979.

Whelan, Elizabeth, *Preventing Cancer*. Norton, 1978.

PERIODICALS

Abram, Morris B., "The Will to Live." *Cancer News*, Spring/Summer 1979.

Adonis, Catherine, "French Cultural Attitudes Towards Cancer." *Cancer Nursing*, April 1978.

Auerbach, Oscar, et al., "Effects of Cigarette Smoking on Dogs: II. Pulmonary Neoplasms." *Archives of Environmental Health*, Vol. 21, December 1970.

Balkwill, Frances, "What Future for the Interferons?" *New Scientist*, January 24, 1980.

Blot, William J., and Joseph F. Fraumeni Jr., "Arsenical Air Pollution and Lung Cancer." *The Lancet*, July 26, 1975.

Cherry, Laurence, "The Brain." *GEO*, October 1980.

Cody, Mrs. James, "The Miracle at St. Jude." *Family Health/Today's Health*, November 1976.

Cole, Philip, and Franco Merletti, "Chemical Agents and Occupational Cancer." *Journal of Environmental Pathology and Toxicology*, 3:399-417, 1980.

"Decision-Making in Cancer Chemotherapy." *Patient Care*, October 15, 1979.

DeVita, Vincent T. and Lorraine M. Kershner, "Cancer, the Curable Diseases." *American Pharmacy*, April 1980.

Epstein, M. A., "Epstein-Barr Virus as the Cause of a Human Cancer." *Nature*, August 24, 1978.

Friedman, Bonnie Denmark, "Coping with Cancer: A Guide for Health Care Professionals." *Cancer Nursing*, April 1980.

Gold, Michael, "The Cells That Would Not Die." *Science 81*, April 28, 1981.

"Guidelines for the Cancer-Related Checkup." *Ca—A Cancer Journal for Clinicians*, July/August 1980.

Hammond, E. Cuyler, et al., "Smoking and Cancer in the United States." *Preventive Medicine*, 9:169-173, 1980.

Henle, Werner, et al., "The Epstein-Barr Virus." *Scientific American*, July 1979.

Hoover, Robert, "Saccharin—Bitter Aftertaste?" *The New England Journal of Medicine*, 302:573-575, 1980.

MacMahon, Brian, et al., "Coffee and Cancer of the Pancreas." *The New England Journal of Medicine*, March 12, 1981.

Mason, Thomas J., and Robert W. Miller, "Cosmic Radiation at High Altitudes and U.S. Cancer Mortality, 1950-1969." *Radiation Research*, 60:302-306, 1974.

"Our Good Friend, Bill Gargan." *Cancer News*, Spring/Summer 1979.

Rosenbaum, Ron, "A Journey Through the Cancer Cure Underground." *New West*, November 17, 1980.

Wald, Nicholas, et al., "Low Serum-vitamin-A and Subsequent Risk of Cancer." *The Lancet*, October 18, 1980.

Wheatley, George M., et al., "The Employment of Persons with a History of Treatment for Cancer." *Cancer*, February 1974.

Wynder, Ernst L., "Dietary Habits and Cancer Epidemiology." *Cancer*, 43:1955-1961, 1979.

OTHER PUBLICATIONS

"The Breast Cancer Digest." National Cancer Institute, April 1979.

"Cancer Facts and Figures 1981." American Cancer Society, 1980.

Hammond, E. Cuyler, and The American Cancer Society, "American Cancer Society Cancer Prevention Study, 1959-1979." American Cancer Society, 1979.

Shiffman, Saul M., and Murray E. Jarvik, "Withdrawal Symptoms: First Week Is Hardest." World Smoking and Health, Winter 1980.

Shimkin, Michael B.: *Contrary to Nature*. U.S. Department of Health, Education and Welfare, 1979. "Science and Cancer." U.S. Department of Health and Human Services, 1980.

U.S. Department of Health, Education and Welfare: "Atlas of Cancer Mortality for U.S. Counties: 1950-1969." Public Health Service/National Institutes of Health, 1975. "Clearing the Air: A Guide to Quitting Smoking." Public Health Service/National Institutes of Health, 1979. *Smoking and Health: A Report of the Surgeon General*. Office on Smoking and Health/Public Health Service, 1971. "The Smoking Digest." Public Health Service/National Institutes of Health, 1977.

Picture credits

The sources for the illustrations in this book appear below. The credits for the illustrations from left to right are separated by semicolons, from top to bottom by dashes.

Cover: Jim Houghton. 7: The Pierpont Morgan Library. 9: Bruce Benedict from Winter Park. 11: Walter E. Hilmers Jr., HJ Commercial Art. 13: Frederic F. Bigio from B-C Graphics. 14: Shinkichi Natori, Tokyo—Charlie Phillips; Brian Brake, New Zealand—E. Schwab from World Health Organization, Geneva. 15: Dr. Nick Day from C.I.R.C., Lyons—E. Schwab from World Health Organization, Geneva. 17: Walter E. Hilmers Jr., HJ Commercial Art. 19, 20: John Tellick, London. 21: John Tellick, London—Charmian Goldwyn, London. 22: Charmian Goldwyn, London. 26-43: Linda Bartlett. 45: Canadian Cancer Society. 47: Manfred Kage from Peter Arnold, Inc. 48: Courtesy National Smoking and Health Association, Stockholm. 51-53: John McDermott. 56: © 1980 Linda Bartlett. 58, 59: Raphael Warshaw; Dr. Irving J. Selikoff, Environmental Sciences Lab, School of Medicine, Dept. of Community Medicine at Mt. Sinai Hospital; Dr. W. Nicholson, Environmental Sciences Lab, School of Medicine, Dept. of Community Medicine at Mt. Sinai Hospital (2). 60, 61: Joan S. McGurren—chart by Walter E. Hilmers Jr., HJ Commercial Art. 63: American Cancer Society. 65-68: Fil Hunter. 69: Fil Hunter—insert, Trudy Nicholson. 71: © 1980 Burt Glinn from Magnum. 73: Georgetown University Hospital. 74, 75: Walter E. Hilmers Jr., HJ Commercial Art. 77: © 1980 Burt Glinn from Magnum—Dr. Dean Jacques from Huntington Institute; Dan McCoy from Rainbow. 78, 79: American Cancer Society; Joan S. McGurren; Memorial Sloan-Kettering Cancer Center (3). 80: Alexander Tsiaras; courtesy Dr. H. Goldstein from University of Pennsylvania. 84: Breitenbach from World Health Organization, Geneva. 86-89: Richard Anderson. 90, 91: Richard Anderson, except inset, Mario A. Grosso, M.D., Georgetown University. 93: Dr. Andrejs Liepins. 94: © 1980 Linda Bartlett. 97-99: Nicholas Fasciano. 101: Dr. Howard Jones Jr.—School of Public Health at the University of California at Berkeley. 105: Dr. Denis Burkitt, St. Thomas' Hospital, London. 106, 107: Trudy Nicholson; Walter E. Hilmers Jr., HJ Commercial Art (2). 108: Margaret Ryon-Uibel. 110-121: Richard Anderson. 123: © 1980 Dan McCoy from Rainbow. 125: Walter E. Hilmers Jr., HJ Commercial Art. 128: © 1980 Howard Sochurek. 131: Dmitri Kessel, courtesy Musée de L'Assistance Publique, Paris. 132: © 1980 Burt Glinn from Magnum, cour-

tesy Bristol-Myers Co.; Dan McCoy from Rainbow. 134: Alexander Tsiaras. 137-140: Peter Barry Chowka. 143: American Cancer Society. 146, 147: James Mason, courtesy American Cancer Society. 149: © 1980 Linda Bartlett; Rutgers University School of Communications. 150: American Cancer Society; Michael Childers; Press Association Ltd., London; Ron Galella—Brack from Black Star; Wide World; Curt Gunther from Camera 5; David Frazier—Henry Groskinsky; © 1976 David Sutton; Wide World; Raeanne Rubenstein—Marion Kaplan; The Washington Redskins; Zoe Dominic, London; Burton Berinsky, courtesy International Creative Management. 152, 153: Derek Bayes, London. 154-157: © 1980 Linda Bartlett. 158: Courtesy The Soviet Cancer Research Center, Moscow—Sovfoto. 159: Tata Memorial Hospital, Parel, Bombay; World Health Organization, Geneva. 160: Masachika Suhara, Tokyo; © 1979 Burt Glinn from Magnum. 161: Photo Vons-Institut Curie, Paris—Ligue Nationale Française contre le Cancer, Paris. 162: Norman Wilson, London; The Institute of Cancer Research and The Royal Marsden Hospital, Sutton, Surrey. 163: Sergio Del Grande/Mondadori, Milan.

Acknowledgments

The index of this book was prepared by Barbara L. Klein. For their help in the preparation of this volume, the editors wish to thank the following: Professor G. E. Adams, Sutton Surrey, England; Sharon Almes, Georgetown University Hospital, Washington, D.C.; American Cancer Society, National Headquarters, New York City; Robert Avery, The Johns Hopkins Oncology Center, Baltimore; Raymond Barmont, Paris; Dr. Renato Baserga, Temple University School of Medicine, Philadelphia; Dr. Z. M. Beekman, Amsterdam; Dr. James Bennett, Albany Medical College, N.Y.; Dr. June L. Biedler, Donald S. Walker Laboratory, Rye, N.Y.; Dr. Ralph Blocksma, Holland, Mich.; Dr. William Blot, National Cancer Institute, Bethesda, Md.; Maryanne Bolton, The Children's Hospital of Philadelphia, Pa.; Helene G. Brown & Associates, Los Angeles; Dr. Denis Burkitt, Gloucestershire, England; Dr. Rebecca L. Byrd, The Children's Hospital of Philadelphia, Pa.; Lois Nelson Callahan, American Cancer Society, Washington, D.C.; Dr. Byungkyn Chun, Georgetown University Hospital, Washington, D.C.; Dr. Olcay Cigtay, Georgetown University Hospital, Washington, D.C.; Sue Cody, Memphis, Tenn.; Dr. Philip Cole, University of Alabama, Bir-

mingham; Jacques des Courtils, Paris; Professor Sir Alastair Currie, University of Edinburgh; Dr. Raymond Damadian, New York City; Dr. Juan A. del Regato, University of South Florida, Tampa; Deutsche Krebshilfe, Bonn; Dr. Vincent T. DeVita Jr., National Cancer Institute, Bethesda, Md.; Professor Stuart Donnan, University of Hong Kong; Dr. Allan Dumont, New York University School of Medicine, New York City; Maggie Duncan, National Hospice Organization, McLean, Va.; Dr. Jean-François Duplan, Bordeaux; Marge DuVall, Georgetown University School of Medicine, Washington, D.C.; Denise Escudier, Paris; Dr. Audrey E. Evans, The Children's Hospital of Philadelphia, Pa.; Lynda Firment, Georgetown University School of Medicine, Washington, D.C.; Lawrence Garfinkel, American Cancer Society, New York City; Marlene Goldman, Harvard School of Public Health, Boston; Dr. Harold A. Goldstein, Hospital of the University of Pennsylvania, Philadelphia; Dr. June Goodfield, Rockefeller University, New York City; Dr. Mario A. Grosso, Georgetown University Hospital, Washington, D.C.; Dr. Jay Harris, Harvard Medical School, Boston; Dr. John Harshbarger, Smithsonian Institution, Washington, D.C.; Dr. Werner Henle, The Children's Hospital of Philadelphia, Pa.; Dr. George Higgins, Veterans Administration Medical Center, Washington, D.C.; Dr. Edwin C. Holstein, Mt. Sinai School of Medicine, New York City; Dr. Michel Hubert-Habart, Institut Curie, Paris; Tom Huisman, Georgetown University Hospital, Washington, D.C.; Dr. Heizaburo Ichikawa, National Cancer Center Hospital, Tokyo; International Union against Cancer, Geneva; Elaine Ipswitch, Fillmore, Calif.; Dr. Shichiro Ishikawa, Japan National Cancer Center, Tokyo; Dr. Dean Jacques, Pasadena, Calif.; Dr. Elaine Jaffe, National Cancer Institute, Bethesda, Md.; A. L. Bud Jones, Golin/-Harris Communications, Inc., Chicago; Ernst Keil, Bonn; Dr. Donald Kerwin, Georgetown University Hospital, Washington, D.C.; Rose Kushner, Kensington, Md.; Martha Laos, Georgetown University Hospital, Washington, D.C.; Professor Raymond Latarjet, Institut Curie, Paris; John Lubera, American Cancer Society, New York City; Dr. Nael Martini, Memorial Sloan-Kettering Cancer Center, New York City; Dr. Thomas J. Mason, National Cancer Institute, Bethesda, Md.; Memorial Sloan-Kettering Cancer Center, Cancer Communications and Public Affairs Departments, New York City; Dr. Wolfgang Mergner, University of Maryland, Baltimore; Dr. H. Metzler, Heidelberg; Dr. Albert R. Milan, Baltimore; Dr. Gerald P. Murphy, Roswell Park Memorial Institute, Buffalo, N.Y.; National Cancer Institute, Office of Cancer Communications, Bethesda, Md.; Dr. Walter Nelson-Rees, University of California, Oakland; Dr. William J. Nicholson, Mt. Sinai School of Medicine, New York City; Dr. Stanley E. Order, The Johns Hopkins Oncology Center, Baltimore; Adele Paroni, American Cancer Society, New York City; George Petrisek, Port Allegheny, Pa.; Captain Philip E. Phelps III, Philadelphia; Dr. John Potter, Georgetown University Hospital, Washington, D.C.; Dr. Alan S. Rabson, National Cancer Institute, Bethesda, Md.; Dr. Lars M. Ramström, National Smoking and Health Association, Stockholm; Dr. Robert W. Rand, University of California, Los Ange-

les; Francine Raymond, Paris; Lucia Roberts, Hospice Care of the District of Columbia, Washington; Dr. Ernest H. Rosenbaum, San Francisco; Dame Cicely Saunders, St. Christopher's Hospice, London; Dr. Joseph F. Saunders, National Cancer Institute, Bethesda, Md.; Dr. George H. Scherr, Pathotox Publishers, Park Forest South, Ill.; Professor Léon Schwartzenberg, Institut Gustave-Roussy, Villejuif, France; Paul Scriffignano, International Association of Laryngectomees, New York City; Dr. Irving J. Selikoff, Mt. Sinai School of Medicine, New York City; Christopher R. Shea, Georgetown University Hospital, Washington, D.C.; Dr. Michael B. Shimkin, La Jolla, Calif.; Susan Silver, Hospice Care of the District of Columbia, Wash-

ington; Hilke Stamiadis-Smidt, Heidelberg; Jeff Teramani, Georgetown University Hospital, Washington, D.C.; Dr. Stuart R. Toledano, The Children's Hospital of Philadelphia, Pa.; U.S.S.R. Cancer Research Center, Moscow; Dr. Moody D. Wharam Jr., The Johns Hopkins Oncology Center, Baltimore; G. Congdon Wood, American Cancer Society, New York City; Professor Umberto Veronesi, Istituto Nazionale Tumori, Milan; Grey Villet, Shushan, N.Y.; Derek Vonberg, London; Dr. John D. Weisburger, Naylor Dana Institute for Disease Prevention, Valhalla, N.Y.; World Health Organization, Geneva; James Young, Arlington Hospital, Va.; Dr. Eva Zinreich, The Johns Hopkins Oncology Center, Baltimore.

Index *Numerals in italics indicate an illustration of the subject mentioned.*

Printed in U.S.A.